VISUAL IMPAIRMENT

Visual Impairment

Ranjita Dawn

KALPAZ

ISBN: 978-93-5128-137-5
Price: ₹ 750/-

First Published, 2015

Published by

Kalpaz Publications
C-30, Satyawati Nagar,
Delhi —110052
E-mail: kalpaz@hotmail.com
Ph.: 9212142040

Laser Typesetting : Rajender Vashist, Delhi
Printed at : G. Print Process, Delhi

Cataloging in Publication Data--DK

Courtesy: D.K. Agencies (P) Ltd. <docinfo@dkagencies.com>

Dawn, Ranjita, author.
Visual impairment / Ranjita Dawn.
pages cm
Includes bibliographical references (pages).
ISBN 9789351281375

1. Vision disorders--India. 2. Students with visual disabilities--India. 3. Students with visual disabilities--Education--India. I. Title.

DDC 362.410954 23

Contents

Acknowledgements 9

Abbreviations 11

List of Tables 13

1. **Understanding Disability** **15**

• Notions and Models of Disability

• Individual Approach of Disability • Criticism of the Individual Approach of Disability • Social Approach of Disability • Criticism of the Social Approach of Disability • Overall Analysis of Notions and Models of Disability

2. **Visual Impairment** **39**

• Blindness

• The Effects of Blindness

• Low Vision

3. **Policies and Perspectives on the Education of People with Disabilities** **49**

• Education of the Disabled: International Scenario

• Special or Residential Schools

• Recent Trends in Non-integrated or Special Education for Disabled Children in India • Residential School Education for Students with Visual Impairment in India

- Integrated Educational Settings: International Scenario

  • Recent Trends in Integrated Education for Children with Disabilities in India • Integrated Education for Students with Visual Impairment in India

- Debate between Non-integrated or Special and Integrated Educational Schools
- Inclusive Education: Quality Education for All

  • Inclusive Education for the Disabled: The Indian Scenario

4. Barriers in the Education of People with Disabilities 69

- Barriers in the Education of Students with Disabilities in India
- Barriers in the Education of Students with Visual Impairment in India

5. Curriculum and Instructional Practices 87

- Facing the Challenge of Curriculum Access and Instructional Practices
- Curriculum and Instructional Practices for Blind Students and Students with Low Vision
- The Core Curriculum for Blind and Visually Impaired Children and Youths

  • Pre-school Blind or Visually Impaired • Curriculum for the Elementary and Secondary Levels • The Existing Core Curriculum • The Expanded Core Curriculum • Significance of the Expanded Core Curriculum for Blind and Visually Impaired Students

- Curriculum Suggestions for Teaching Students with Low Vision

  • Teaching of Mathematics • Language teaching • Teaching of Social Studies • Teaching of

Science • Unique Curriculum Needs for Students with Low Vision

- Curriculum Suggestions for Teaching Students with Visual Impairment and Other Disabilities
- Instructional Practices for Students with Visual Impairments and Developmental Disabilities

6. Assistive Technology 105

- Role of Assistive Technology for Blind Students and Students with Low Vision
- Non-electronic Equipment
- Advent and Evolution of Braille in India
- Electronic Equipment
- Orientation and Mobility Aids
- Issues and Challenges
- Implications for Practice
- Conclusion

7. Teachers: Aproach, Attitudes and Roles 121

- Teachers Role and Approach
- Suggestions for Teachers of Students who are Blind or Visually Impaired

8. Accessibility and Infrastructure for Persons with Disabilities in India 129

- Initiatives
- Conclusion

9. Issues and Challenges in the Employment of Persons with Disabilities in India 139

- Critical Review of the Policies and the Legislation Process
- Suggestive Measures
- Conclusion

10. Rehabilitative Services 149

11. Conclusion **163**

Bibliography 167

Appendices 177

Appendix A: Developmental Milestones for Infants with Visual Impairments

Appendix B: Checklist for the Teachers for Observation of Symptoms that may Indicate a Visual Problem

Appendix C: Eye Conditions

Appendix D: Medical Certificate: Vision

Appendix E: File Review Form

Appendix F: Interview with Parents

Appendix G: Information from an Education Consultant or Itinerant

Index 231

Acknowledgements

At the very outset a special word of appreciation for my family members. There are no words sufficient enough to express love and gratitude for my family members—my mother, my sister, my brother and my son, Sachdeep, for their tremendous support. I would like to thank them for standing by me throughout my life and for everything they all have done for me. This book would never have materialised without their love, presence and sacrifices.

I extend my sincere gratitude to each and every one for the rich experiences they have given me which enabled me to undertake this work and complete it.

I also extend my gratitude to the M/s Kalpaz Publications, New Delhi for undertaking the publication of the work.

Ranjita Dawn

Acknowledgements

Abbreviations

CRPD	Convention on Rights of Persons with Disabilities.
CWD	Children With Disabilities.
DDRC	District Disability and Rehabilitation Centres.
DFID	Department for International Development.
DISE	District Information System for Education.
DPEP	District Primary Education Programme.
EFA	Education for All.
ICDS	Integrated Child Development Services.
ICIDH	International Classification of Impairments, Disabilities, and Handicaps.
IECYD	Inclusion in Education of Children and Youth with Disabilities.
IEDC	Integrated Education for the Disabled Children.
IEDSS	Inclusive Education of the Disabled at the Secondary Stage.
MHRD	Ministry of Human Resource and Development.
NAB	The National Association for the Blind.
NCERT	National Council for Educational Research and Training.
NCPEDP	National Centre for Promotion of Employment for Disabled People.
NGO	Non-Government Organisation.
NPE	National Policy of Education.

NSSO	National Sample Survey Organisation.
PIED	Projected Integrated Education for the Disabled.
PWD	Persons with Disabilities Act, 1995.
RCI	Rehabilitation Council of India.
RTI	Response to Intervention Model.
SSA	Sarva Shiksha Abhiyan.
UN	United Nations.
UNDP	United Nations Development Programme.
UNESCO	United Nations Educational, Scientific and Cultural Organisation.
UNICEF	United Nations Children's Education Fund.
UPIAS	Union of the Physically Impaired Against Segregation.
WHO	World Health Organisation.

List of Tables

1.1 Handicap as Conceptualised within Different Systems 33

1.2 Comprehensive Picture of the Shifting Paradigms of the Social Approach of Disability 35

1.3 Differences between the Medical and Social Models 37

2.1 Prevalence and Incidence of Visually Disabled Persons per 1,00,000 Persons 43

2.2 NSSO Report—Prevalence of Visual Disability 44

2.3 Age Group and Visual Impairment 44

2.4 Age at the Onset of Visual Disability 45

2.5 Distribution of Blind Persons per 1,000 by Cause of Blindness Sex-wise and Sector-wise—All India 46

2.6 Per 1000 Distribution of Persons with Low Vision by Cause of Low Vision for Each Sex and Sector—All-India 46

4.1 Identification of CWSN 73

4.2 Enrolment According to the Type of Disability 74

4.3 Enrollment of Disabled Children in Schools under the Integrated Educational Programme (Stage: Primary) 78

4.4 Enrollment of Disabled Children in Schools under the Integrated Educational Programme (Stage: Upper Primary) 78

4.5 Distribution of Aids and Appliances 80

8.1 Percentage of People with Disabilities Affected by Various Aspects of Pedestrian Environment 132

8.2 Continuum of Necessary Interventions for Countries to Make their Transport Systems Accessible for all 136

9.1 Performance of the Special Employment Exchange for Persons with Disabilities in 1999 140

9.2 Employment Rates of Persons with Disabilities by State/Union Territory 141

9.3 Reserved Posts for PWD Identified and Filled, Early 2000s 143

9.4 PWD placed by employment exchanges (in thousands) 144

9.5 Distribution of Working Age Persons with Disabilities by Usual Activity Status (15 to 64 years) in 2002 146

1

Understanding Disability

The inherent tendency of human beings to give meanings to objects in the social world and subsequently to orientate their behaviour towards these objects in terms of the meanings given to them is the origin of the fundamental difference between a social world and the natural world. As far as disability is concerned, it, too, has been variously defined from being a deficit, exclusion, a deviation from the norm, disadvantage, social oppression, a collection of barriers, a challenge, an experience, an identity, a process to a predicament, difference, an aspect of diversity, and at one end of a continuum with health. In relation to this, the Department for International Development (DFID) white paper on disability and development specified that 'defining disability is complicated – and controversial' (2000:2). Albert (2004) also identified the need to more clearly conceptualise disability in the field of international development because how disability is explained points to the location of action to address associated injustice. Hence, theoretical claims and debates about the nature of disability are predominantly characterised by perspectives that conceive of mind, body, and society as separate spheres of human existence. In particular, disability theory tends to revolve around the dichotomy of individual/medical and social conceptions of disability.

Notions and Models of Disability

Discourses of disability are characterised by a myriad of competing and often conflicting viewpoints on the nature and determinants of disability. A major focuss for these debates has centred on the issue of definitions of disability and these, therefore, have consequently undergone a number of changes and modifications. These range from Western biomedical discourses (Rhodes, 1985), which conceive of disability as a state of dysfunctioning body parts, to social perspectives which see disability as society's denial of opportunities to those with impairment (Oliver, 1990). Between these extremes, a range of views is evident, including perspectives which regard disability as a form of social deviance (Goffman, 1963), to traditions within social psychology that emphasise the interactive nature of disability (Safilos-Rothschild, 1970). More recently, post-modern and post-structuralist discourses, which conceive of disability as a series of socio-cultural constructions, have gained some ascendancy (Butler, 1993; Paterson and Hughes, 1999).

Individual Approach of Disability

The Individual approach often referred to as 'personal tragedy theory' views the problems faced by disabled people as having directly emanated due to individual dysfunction. The individual approach encompasses two models within its broad framework—the Medical model and the Psychological model.

The Medical Model emanated from the disease model of medicine, which predisposes practitioners to think of a 'condition' that needs appropriate treatment. It is believed that the Medical model appeared as a consequence of the WHO (1980) debate on usefulness of terms such as 'handicap', 'impairment' and 'disability'. According to it, disability came to be defined as the effect of impairment on everyday activities thereby reducing the origins of disability to individual pathology. This paradigm makes two fundamental assumptions—it locates the problem of disability within the individual and seeks the cause of the problem as stemming from functional limitations that arise from disability (Fig 1.1). The human being under such circumstances is viewed as flexible and alterable as compared to the fixed and unalterable society. Disability under this approach was not regarded as a defining state wherein disabling conditions such as 'mental retardation', 'blindness', etc., were taken into consideration along with other conditions that were not capable of causing disabilities. Emphasising on individual pathology or biological determinism, the model holds that all differences can be wiped with prostheses, exercises, medical interventions and by stimulating disabled people to adapt to the norms.

Disabled People as Passive Receivers of Services Aimed at Cure or Management

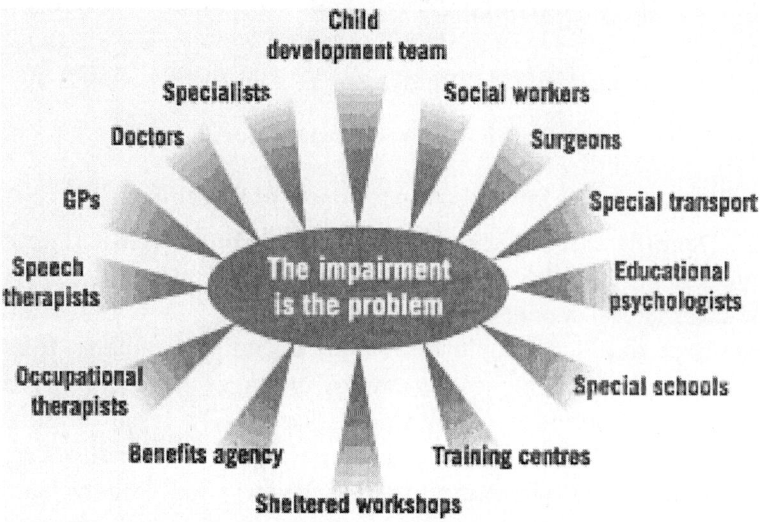

Fig 1.1. The Medical Model .

The Psychological Model focussed on the use of clinical diagnostic criteria like 'standardised measures' for assessing, quantifying the problems, categorising and labelling individuals. It negates the realisation that disability emanates from social situation such as barriers of environment and attitude of an individual with an impairment or functional limitation. It upholds the assumption that all people with impairments are automatically handicapped or handicap their family and that the society has not been constructed to include disabled people and make provisions for this diversity (Fig 1.2).

Model of Shared Psychobiological Pathways

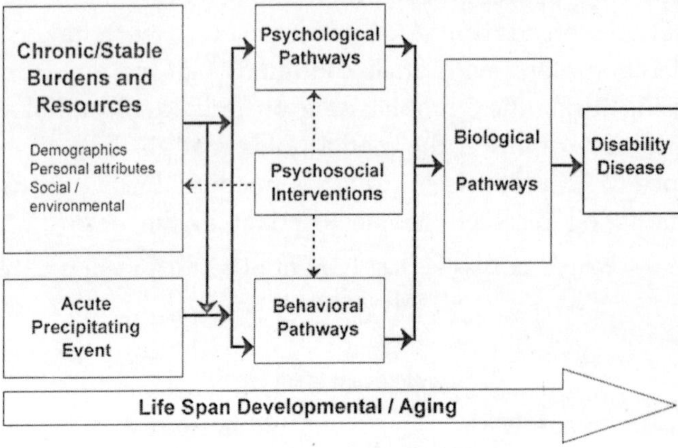

Fig 1.2: The Psychological Model.

Criticism of the Individual Approach of Disability

Despite the numerous arguments, both Medical and Psychological models were subjected to severe criticism. Critiques of the Medical model opined that it failed to take into account views of disabled people for whom disability emanates from the society's unwillingness to employ and alter necessary means rather than individual dysfunction. The WHO's (1980) original classification, the International Classification of Impairments, Disabilities, and Handicaps (ICIDH), which has largely been discredited for its medical tenor and for focussing on the limitations of people's abilities as the key determinant of disability. The ICIDH is problematical because it fails to 'acknowledge the presence of social barriers' in influencing disability.

In simplest terms, the Medical model assumes that the first step solution is to find a cure or to use WHO terminology, i.e., make disabled people more 'normal'. This invariably fails because disabled people are not necessarily sick or cannot be improved by remedial treatment. The only remaining solution is to accept the 'abnormality' and provide the necessary care to support the 'incurable' impaired person. Policy makers are limited to a range of options based upon a programme of rehabilitation, vocational training for employment, income maintenance programs and the provision of aids and equipment.

On the contrary, the Medical model regarded them as objects without power and incapable of managing their own lives. It also failed to realise that although medical conditions restricted the functioning of people with disabilities which may or may not have required medical treatment, human knowledge, technology and collective resources did not prevent them from experiencing good lives.

The essence of the Medical model which reduces identity of the disabled to that of deviants, damaged, dependent carriers of sick role and perpetuating labels subjecting them to continuous stigmatisation and marginalisation can be best summed up in the following lines:

'The injunction to be particular sort of person is always bound up with an act of division: to be what one is, one must be what one is not... The vicissitudes of identification are not ontological but historical and technical' (Rose, 1996, p. 309).

The impositions of medically defined and adult imposed notions of difference and normality to the identity of disabled in terms of labels are also evident in both 'special' and 'mainstream' settings whereby children are expected to comply with the definition and status imposed on them. Stambolvic (1996) and Camilleri (1999) also criticised the Medical model for portraying the needs of disabled people as special and different from others thereby reducing disability to personal tragedy, highlighting the inabilities, overlooking the latent abilities of disabled people and promoting human helplessness.

With marked emphasis on the use of clinical diagnostic criteria such as standardised measures of intelligence or self-concept to identify the nature of the problem, critiques maintained that the psychological model posed certain hindrances. Worthen and Spandel (1991) maintained that the tests used had little association with learning and low predictive value resulting in categorisation and labelling of children. Llewellyn and Chung (1997) also questioned the authenticity of measures associated with identifying and segregating what is 'normal' in the sphere of disability research.

The Individual approach to disability has been subjected to severe criticism for its narrow and reductionist nature and failure to consider the significance of psychological and sociological causes resulting in disabling conditions. Moreover, this approach was also found to play a dominant role in making individuals feel receptive, passive and compliant thus promoting human helplessness. The model imposes a paternalistic approach to problem solving which, although well intentioned, concentrates on 'care' and ultimately provides justification for institutionalisation and segregation. This restricts disabled people's opportunities to make choices, control their lives and develop their potential. The above arguments necessitated the need for a paradigm shift in the area of disability studies. This assumed a form with the formulation and acceptance of Social approach of disability.

Social Approach of Disability

The issue of disability has been historically conceptualised by different disciplines such as sociology and social policy using a range of theoretical approaches. Before critical analysing the social approach of disability, it is essential to look into the background that caused its foundation. Several sociological accounts have been shaped by the Parsonian paradigm according to which people with disabilities authorise medical professionals to undertake the shaping of their lives thus alleviating them from their 'abhorrent and undesirable situation' (Parsons, 1951). Parsons (1951) adopted a functional approach to health and illness treating illness as a social role with precise expectations and limitations. According to him, sickness exempted people with disabilities from the obligations and responsibilities that other members of society undertook thereby characterising them in terms of 'incapacity' and 'deviance'. Parsons opined that conformity to 'normal' social roles facilitated in maintaining the integrity of social systems. Early works in disability research based on the Parsonian perspective show that maintenance of social system being the prime focuss made it imperative for all members of the society to execute their appropriate social roles.

Later a shift in paradigm subjected the Parsonian perspective to severe criticism. It was argued that although Parson's viewpoints were more suitable for impairments that were acute and transitory in nature its implication was not suitable on those which were permanent or chronic in nature. Some researchers further maintained that it was possible for the sick or impaired individuals to recover function or health within the context of their life position and resources since the meanings associated with them are conditioned by one's position and the socials group to which they belong (Kassebaum and Baumann, 1965; Gordon, 1973). Critically analysing the Parsonian paradigm—Twaddle (1974) pointed out that while emphasising on social and psychological reality of disease, it failed to take into consideration the organic base of illness.

Another viewpoint that emerged regarding disability studies was the Deviance approach. The deviance theorists viewed people with disabilities as 'being deviant' from others. Goffman (1963) visualised the abnormal nature of people with disabilities as a source of stigma among the non-disabled which marked them as different and harmful. Friedson (1965) also visualised people with disabilities as social deviants. According to him, identification of factors that brings some people in conflict with society's morals and values facilitate the changes required for them to be accepted by the non disabled. He thereby emphasised on deviance by using the term in the context of institution.

Later, the deviance model was subjected to severe criticism. Haber and Smith (1971) rejected the model based on the argument that the key to the disabled role lay with legitimation whereby the external behaviour of disabled individuals were normalised through mechanisms that provided new social meanings and rules of interaction for persons with disabilities.

A marked change was observed in the field of disability research with the coming of the Social approach. Under this approach, disability came to be conceptualised as an interaction between individual and society. It argued that whether a person was being labeled as disabled primarily depended on how the society arranged circumstances in order to compensate for the individual impairments. The articulation of this new view of disability did not receive universal acceptance. Originally, it was professionals, policy makers and staff from organisations for disabled people who questioned the experiential validity and explanatory reliability of the social model since they had vested interests in maintaining the status quo underpinned by the individual model. Later, a paradigm shift was evident as many professional bodies and groups advocated the social model, in theory at least (DHSS 1988; Gillespie-Sells and Campbell, 1991). The social model was received more enthusiastically by people with disabilities themselves as it fostered immediate connection with their own experiences.

The arguments of the social approach were well reflected in the earlier works of UPIAS (Union of the Physically Impaired Against Segregation, 1976) which defined disability as 'the disadvantage or restriction of activities caused by contemporary social organisations and thus takes little or no account of people with physical impairment and thus excludes them from participating in the mainstream of social activities' (Fig 1.3).

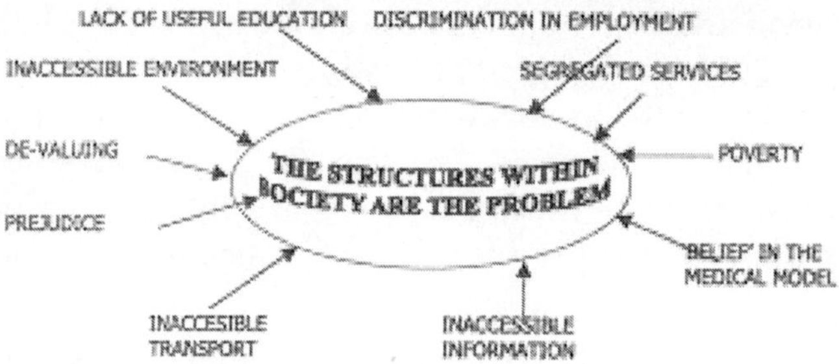

Disables People as Active Fighters for Equality Working in Partnership with Allies

Fig 1.3: Social Model

The earliest attempt to concretise the social approach was made by Mike Oliver with the view to reflect the growing distress and demands of people with disabilities and their allies for 'nothing more fundamental than a switch away from focussing on the physical limitations of particular individuals to the way the physical and social environments impose on certain groups or categories of people' (Oliver, 1983:23).

According to Oliver, the Social approach does not deny the problem of disability but locates it within the society. Failure on the part of society to take into account the needs of people with disabilities and provide appropriate services to them rather than the individual limitations promotes the problem. Oliver (1996) opined that the 'impaired' or 'disabled' role makes individuals 'accept dependency', and make most of their abilities to achieve ' normality'. The oppression that people with disabilities face in the society results from institutional discrimination 'ranging from individual prejudice to institutional discrimination, from inaccessible public buildings to unusable transport system, from segregated education to excluding work arrangements and so on (Oliver 1996:33). According to him, lack of mobility is impairment, but lack of access to essential facilities was disability.

The Social approach also regarded as 'Social Oppression Theory' includes within it two perspectives on disability—Social Constructivist and Social-Creationist. Besides these two broad perspectives, the social approach encompasses a number of other theoretical perspectives: Functionalism, Conflict, Interactionism and Post-modernism which would be critically discussed in the forthcoming section. The two other sub-models that can be discussed within the framework of the Social approach of disability are the Systems model and the Transactional model.

The Social-Constructivists view disability as a problem located within the minds of able-bodied people, whether individually (prejudice) or collectively, through the manifestation of hostile social attitudes and enactment of social policies based upon a tragic view of disability. This approach holds that individuals become a part of the existing world only when they learn and acquire socially anchored values and beliefs. The various meanings that people learn to attach to various activities have an impact on their ability to interact with the environment. Similarly, disability for them is defined by the meaning that we attach to different kinds of physical and mental deviations.

Researchers like Rose (1962) held that disability is only in a particular and narrowest sense a condition that a person has. The word disability (and the many subcategories under the heading) does not simply symbolise a condition that is already there in advance, it makes possible the existence or appearance of the condition for it is part of the mechanism. Hence, they held that as a concept disability is a particular way of thinking, acting and reacting while the creation of disability concept, its application in specific settings and the effect it provokes is derived from and sustained in interaction. The most common means that are associated and results in segregation of disabled individuals from mainstream society are the effects of categorisation, labelling and institutionalisation. The labelling and categorisation of an individual as 'disabled' puts the person in a category that is loaded with social meanings and preconceptions. The treatment that individuals receive from significant others in the society causes them to internalise the image inherent in labels. This in turn determines their behaviour pattern and affects their self-image.

Under the Social-Constructivist approach, Soder (1989) outlined two other ways of viewing the relation between disability and environment—(a) Epidemiological approach and (b) Adaptability approach. The Epidemiological approach viewed disability as a disturbance within an individual with environment being treated as the potential cause of disturbances. This approach seeks to describe as well as interpret the distribution of disabilities within different substratas of a population and locate it in a geographical and social structure in causal terms. On the other hand, the Adaptability approach regarded disability as an outcome of interaction between individual and environment rather than an intrinsic personal characteristic or abnormality within an individual. Hence, according to the Social—Constructivists, environment 'is seen as the creator of disability' (Soder, 1989).

The Social Creationists (Abberley, 1987; Oliver, 1992) perceived disability not as something that exists within the minds of individuals or groups or even society as a whole but in the institutionalised practices of the society. According to them, impairment is not an unavoidable 'fact of nature' but is primarily the consequence of social and political factors such as malnutrition, drug abuse, lack of medical treatment (Abberley, 1987). Abberley (1987) opined that besides emphasising on the deplorable state of people with disabilities, there is the need to develop a more comprehensive theoretical approach which would facilitate masses to understand that perception of people with disabilities as 'disabled' are dialectically related to an ideology or a group of ideologies that further perpetuates the existing situation.

Among the other theoretical perspectives included within the Social approach of disability are: Functionalism, Conflict, Interactionism and Post-modernism. The earliest theory of functionalism was evident in the sociological works of Emile Durkheim. Durkheim (1964) posited a fundamental difference between pre-industrial and industrial societies. According to him, social integration in the pre-industrial societies was based on similarities of roles in the social division of labour, i.e., 'mechanical solidarity'. However, with the emergence of industrialisation and its continuous emphasis on growing separateness and distinction of an individual from the group due to division of labour, a good society came to be recognised by its strong bonds of 'organic solidarity' that were constituted through the recognition of role of others in the complex division of society. The deprivation of such a role was referred to as deprivation of full societal membership.

The Functional perspective which explains the existence of a phenomenon or execution of an action in terms of its consequences thus contributing towards maintaining a stable whole laid emphasis on order, stability, consensus and maintenance of the *status quo*. Farber referred to the disabled and deviants as 'the surplus population, i.e., a residual population from which recruitment could be made for various positions in the social organisation. By addressing the disabled as a residual population, he regarded people with disabilities as deviants who are unable to adjust and meet the demands of the social setting in which they live and were hence subjected to classification, regulation and treatment. He held that placing them outside the larger society facilitated maintenance of order and stability in the society (cited in Tomlinson, 1984: 14). Such an objective necessitates the need to help children with special needs to adjust to the society by differentiating their needs and allocating them to segregated/separate settings. This was an essential prerequisite for maintenance of social order without the disabled people disturbing the regular educational system.

Emphasising on the viewpoints of Durkheim, Topliss (1982) provided further support for the discrimination against people with disabilities. He maintained that although the type of impairment that disables a person from participating in the society may undergo a change, an inevitable line of distinction continues to remain between the disabled minority and the able bodied majority wherein the interests of the former are given less salience in the activities of the society. In addition to this, continuous emphasis on vigorous independence, competitive achievement in the occupational sphere further facilitates negative and stigmatising view of the disabled. In view of the diverse values which underpines the varied spheres of society aiming to create desired categories of people, people with disabilities are subjected to further stigmatisation and neglect resulting from the 'disablement' which handicap them. Hence, according to Topliss, the inevitable disadvantage of the people with disabilities stems from general inability to meet standards of performance at work.

Emphasising on social control, the Conflict perspective focusses on power and domination of one group over another. It views people with disabilities as a vulnerable group, oppressed and controlled by the larger population, i.e., the so called 'normal' people, who exclude them from the mainstream activities. According to this perspective, people with disabilities assert control over their lives by acting as a group to bring in changes in their disabling environment through laws and policies and altering the attitude of the people towards them through active participation in public life. This marked a shift in emphasis from the Medical model which focussed on functional impairment and the economic model which emphasised on vocational limitations to a Political approach that helped to visualise the problems of people with disabilities resulting from a disabling environment rather than personal limitations. It also encouraged them to take control of the dysfunctional and interpretative processes with the aim of establishing their identities.

Within the context of the Conflict perspective of disability mention can be made of the Human Rights Approach. Burgdorf (1980), Quinn (1995), Degener and Koster-Dreeser (1995) and Seighart (1985) were among the protagonists of this approach to disability. They were of the opinion that people with disabilities possess the same needs as the rest of humanity. The approach advocated for the formulation and implementation of legislation so as to provide leverage towards promoting mainstreaming of the disadvantaged individuals.

However, the critiques of the conflict perspective maintained that while the conflict perspective focussed on the dimensions of conflict, coercion or the vested interests of the disabled in society, it failed to consider the implications and impact that social interaction and the construction of meanings have had on their lives.

Interaction with others holds the focuss of arguments for the Interactionist perspective. The role of 'significant others' which Scott (1999) referred to as 'those people who have the greatest influence on an individual's evaluation of himself and who have the greatest impact on his acceptance and rejection of social norms', facilitates the manner in which people with disabilities give shape to their 'self'. Further, support to the role of significant others in the formation of an identity of self was provided by Cooley (19092) and Mead (1934). Cooley (1902) maintained that an individual develops his conception of the self by way of imagining what others think of him by way of a 'looking glass' process. Later expanding upon Cooley's looking-glass self, Mead (1934) held that self-concept arises in social interaction as an outgrowth of an individual's concern about others reaction to him or her. The need to anticipate others reaction can cause an individual to behave accordingly thereby perceiving the world as the 'others'. Hence Mead (1934) also emphasised on the aspect of self being social and held that an individual comes to know about himself or herself by role playing.

However, the nature of interaction could extend from one of acceptance and compassion to labelling and stigmatisation.

Referring to the concept of stigma, Goffman (1969) maintained that the physically impaired, those with mental disorder, homosexuals and members of racial and religious minorities are viewed by the society as 'not quite human' but as deviants from the 'anticipated norms' (Vernon, 1999). The stigma attributed brings along with it certain negative connotation that prevents individuals with disabilities from being treated at par with their non-disabled counterparts. In the classroom situation also, effective social interaction in terms of ability to reciprocate to others, actions affect the 'concept of self' of children. Labeling further results in self-fulfilling prophecy and prevents the child from realising his or her potential.

The rise of Post-modernism challenged the existence of ultimate truth which could be discovered through reason and rationality. It also marked an end to the dominant beliefs of the Western culture for which world could be understood in terms of the underlying structures such as the economic structure as exemplified in the works of Marx and the psychic structures of Piaget and Freud. The tenets of post-modernism emphasise that there cannot be 'pure' measures of people's contexts and characteristics in order to inevitably arrive at 'purity' as they reflect the distorting practice of filtering out the normal social context of a person's life. According to them, this can be of immense relevance for contemporary research in human behaviour.

The Post-modernist perspective was later applied to the study of disability as an attempt to develop a radical sociology of impairment. Post-modernists like Foucault (1973) attempted to study the power exercised by 'normal' people over people with disabilities. Modernity, according to them, had a pervasive capacity to produce strangers. The limits of tolerance and conformity provided the basis for constructing the aspects of strangeness, while modernity lends support to homogenise and annihilate the differences it invariably produces. The two major viewpoints existing in the generic construction of stranger in modernity regarding people with disabilities are the Anthropophagic (assimilationist) strategy by way of the segregationist policies and the Anthropoemic (exclusionary) strategy by way of community care. However, both the strategies were an outcome of powerful 'ill to order', according to which impairment is constituted in terms of invalidation.

According to Foucault (1973), the stranger produced resulted due to categorisation and normalisation of the propensities of knowledge. For him, the 'gaze' manifests itself more in institutional forms of domination and regulation rather than the oppressiveness of intercorporal relationships. Self-surveillance by which people develop an awareness of how they are through the gaze of others and then modify their behaviour affects both disabled and non-disabled people. Under such circumstances, people with disabilities are subjected to oppression wherein they internalise the prejudices and assumptions held by their non-disabled counterparts. Foucault (1971, 1976) held that medicine and psychoanalysis in addition to the penal system provide examples of disciplinary and regulatory control leading to the criterion of new norms. It is diffusion of the medical discourse that has enabled the Medical model view of disability to become widespread at all levels of the society, affecting the manner in which institutions from the government to industry treat disabled people (Chadwick, 1996). In this relation, 'normal' people use the power of fixing which Sartre (1958) referred to as 'gaze' on the disabled people for not conforming to what they consider 'valid' behaviour.

Sartre (1958) was concerned with the dialectical play of power which manifests itself in the form of 'gaze' of others that subject one to objectification and internalisation. The gaze for him was a 'constituent power', i.e., the power to fix an identity or to 'condemn' an individual identity wherein the absolute freedom of the solipsistic self is displaced by spatialisation and temporisation. In other words the experience of being looked at by others indicates denial of 'transcendence' and transformation into a 'degraded consciousness'. This is also applicable in case of the disabled where the 'steady and corrosive gaze' of the non-disabled others institutionalised in medicine highlights the corporeality of 'truth' and 'perfection' of normality subjects and stigmatises the impaired for lack of wholeness, coherence and unity. Sartre (1982) referred to this gaze in the 'Critique of

Dialectical Reason' as the 'praxis of oppression' which is socially constructed and through which the disabled people experience an act of 'invalidation', being reduced to status of an object itself and condemned to an 'identity'.

The concept of 'gaze' whereby the disabled are placed under constant surveillance of others was also emphasised by Allan (1998). He analysed the formation of children's identities through three mechanisms of surveillance earlier identified by Foucault. He held that from the perspective of Hierarchical Observation one tends to see everything perfectly. According to him, children with special education needs are placed under constant surveillance of those who are entrusted with their supervision wherein the teachers, parents, head teachers and specialists are caught within the network of the gaze. This is chiefly based on the rationale that surveillance of pupils with special education need enable the professionals to show concern for the welfare of such children and acquire knowledge about their disability. At the same time, it also allows the aspect of power or control to remain inherent in the situation as they can enforce their perception of the situation on the children.

Among the other aspects that subject children with special needs to surveillance are the perspective of Normalising Judgements which separates children with special needs from the normal children and the perspective of Examination which tends to objectify the individual by classifying them and labelling them as cases who need to be 'trained or corrected, classified, normalised, excluded, etc.' (Foucault, 1981). The completion of the assessment procedure ensures further subjection of the child and his or her parents to surveillance for the entire school life.

Expanding on the concept of gaze and its impact, Fox (1993) maintained that it was clearly evident in institutional settings where bodies are disciplined. According to him, the body becomes a site of power or knowledge for the disabled people who are constantly under the surveillance of medical experts who use clinical gaze to identify deviance and disorder and to constitute them as patients.

Finkelstein (1980) based on his own experiences and those

of other people with disabilities held that for centuries able bodied people have made decisions for the disabled ranging from deciding on appropriate behaviour pattern for them by means of rehabilitation programme to designing equipments for them with assumed expertise. This resulted in depriving people with disabilities the right to question the objectivity of the able bodied for making decisions on their behalf. He referred to this as the Social Barriers model of disability according to which disability results due to social and attitudinal barriers constructed by a world built for the able bodied. According to Finkelstein, the construction of boundaries among the able bodied and people with disabilities are also handicapped by discipline. Disability, according to him, failed to hold the focuss as a subject or course of study other than remaining as an issue of discussion and a result of human malfunction.

French (1993, 1999, 2001) also emphasised on the role played by the society in disabling blind people using the prior social model of disability literature. She argued that conflicting discourse resulted due to sighted people definition of 'acceptable' and 'normal' behaviour for the visually disabled people and using them to 'contest that person's identity'.

Emphasising on the lack of adequate academic attention to disability studies, Barnes (1999) held that current presentation of 'disability' in the universities fosters the notion that disability is an individual or a family 'problem'. According to her, the absence of 'disabled voice' in the curriculum and shortage of disabled scholars and researchers within the universities largely accounted for inadequate interventions leading to the marginalisation of 'disability' in humanities and liberal arts.

According to Finkelstein, the term 'disabled' or 'abnormal' denoted ownership of particular impairment and signified health problem of the able bodied whereby the disabled were regarded as able bodied victims of the inequities imprisoned in imperfect bodies. This ignorance about the nature of disability characterised the whole residential institutional approach. According to Finkelstein (1980), there have been three phases of development regarding the perception of people with disabilities. In phase one, the disabled people formed a part of a mainstream oppressed underclass. In phase two, the coming of industrialisation, urbanisation, regulation and externalisation of working practices with the rise of capitalism prevented many people with disabilities from keeping pace with the new market economy. This resulted in them being redefined as passive and dependent and segregated from mainstream society to workhouses and asylums. In the third phase, introduction of new technology led to the belief that individual people would help people with impairments to reintegrate into the mainstream society and cause disability to disappear.

Michalko (1998), a post-modern sociologist deconstructed medical, psychological and societal ideas and practices around blindness. In his *'Mystery of the Eye and Shadow of Blindness'* (1998), he critically analysed blindness rehabilitation. He wrote 'Ophthalmology is recommending agency as an actor presented as qualified to speak about, and act upon, permanent blindness...'. He criticised the authority assumed by the medical personnel in diagnosing blind individuals and referring them for rehabilitation. Such an approach suggests that blindness requires an agency and needs to be acted upon for rehabilitation for a 'good life'. In another book, *'The Two in One: Walking with Smokie, Walking with Blindness'*, Michalko analysed his own experience of vision loss and acquisition of a guide dog. He described his personal experience in the living world built by and for the sighted people by using post-colonial concepts of 'home' and 'exile'. He also examined how the dog guide school created expectations about the behaviour of blind students and school environment based on sighted notions about blindness experience.

The Systems model considers the society as a compound of different systems characterised by communication in contrast to the biological systems. It holds that behaviour of human beings can be understood within the perspective of these different systems that are distinct from one another. Bronfenbrenner (1979, 1989), Hayes (1994), Hornby (1994) and Mitchell (1986) were among the leading exponents of the Systems model. According to the Systems model, disability is regarded as a phenomenon that cannot be analysed other than in relation to the distinctive system/environment as individuals do not belong to a system but are a part of the environment. It refers to communication in functionally differentiated systems of the difference between impairment and no impairment. Each system indicates specific codification, whereby individuals are observed in different ways in different systems. The system ascribes a specific coordination to each individual thereby attaching a meaning to the particular individual's condition. All the other aspects of the person are ignored except those that fit the system-specific form of communication. Table 1.1 shows distinctions about handicap as used within different systems.

Table 1.1: Handicap as Conceptualised within Different Systems

Perspectives	*Observation of Disability*
Medical System	Diseases, defects, malfunctions, impairments, treatment
Economic System	Lack of economic resources, inability to pay, poverty
Labour market System	Working disability, inability to engage in gainful activity
Legal System	Legal incapacity, lack of rights/duties
Rehabilitation System	Support/correction of functional incapacities
Education System	Learning difficulties, low education level
Art System	Ugliness, defective body

Source: Oliver (1995).

The basic theoretical underpinning of the approach that behaviour of people with disabilities cannot be considered independent of the social milieu is best demonstrated by the four levels of social systems as shown in Fig 1.4.

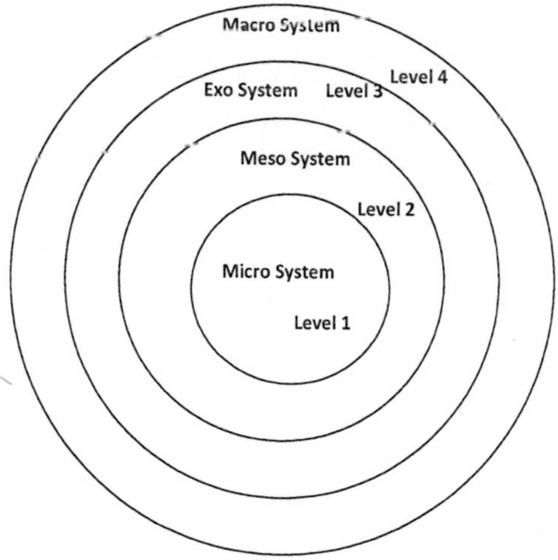

Fig 1.4: Four Levels of Social Systems Based on the Systems Model.

The four levels of social systems include—

- The microsystem including the family and its various subsystems;
- The mesosystem including extended family, friends and neighbours, associates, local agencies participative in delivering services to the disabled individuals;
- The mesosytem is in turn embedded in an exosystem incorporated within which are health, employment, education, social welfare, recreation, voluntary societies and mass media systems'; and
- The macrosystem comprises of the broad values and ideologies of the society.

In accordance with the Systems approach, Bronfenbrenner (1979) maintained that the characteristics of a person at a given time in his or her life are a joint function of the characteristics of the person and the environment till his or her life up to the present time. It emphasised on the need to observe young people with physical disabilities in different contexts and environment at different points of time before making clinical or psychological judgement. Besides this, there is also the need to interpret the assessment of the competencies of any person with disability in the light of the culture or sub-culture in which he or she has been brought up.

In keeping with the above arguments, the advocates of the systems model maintain that the planning, management and evaluation of services for the people with disabilities and their families must address the changing developmental needs of such disadvantaged.

The Transactional Model emphasised on the need to understand the environment as an interactive structure and view individuals as active synthesisers of information from the environment. This was considered to be imperative in understanding the impact that the perceptions of significant others have on the development of persons with disabilities.

Table 1.2: Comprehensive Picture of the Shifting Paradigms of the Social Approach of Disability

Ways of Understanding	*Old Paradigm*	*Alternative 1 (others)*	*Alternative 2 (Oliver)*
Sociological Theory	(Personal Tragedy)	Socio-Political	Political Economy
	Functionalism	Political Economy (Pluralist)	(Materialist)
Middle Range Theorising	Interactionism	Post-Modernism Individual Rights	Social Adjustment
	Adjustment/Loss		
Methodology	Sick Role	Integration	Inclusion
	Deviance/stigma	Personal empowerment	Collective empowerment Emancipatory
	Positivist Interpretive	Participatory Applied research Action research	

Source: Barnes (1995).

Criticism of the Social Approach of Disability

The Social approach of disability has been subjected to certain criticisms. It is held by some researchers that disability exists only in the attitudes or as a function of the social power to coerce which is detrimental. According to them, complete acceptance of the belief that disability is a socially constructed phenomenon might result in regarding disability as 'unreal'. In addition to this misinterpretation of the Social model by some disability activists have resulted in the belief that the model precludes discussions of impairments, importance of 'medical' treatments, ignores the question of gender, minority ethnic status, sexuality, class and so on.

Moreover, constant and increasing emphasis on 'post' theorising has caused a marked shift in focuss to personal narratives and experiences (Hughes and Paterson, 1997; Shakespeare, 1997) and analysis of role of impairment in the process of disablement. The diverse discourse on Social model has diluted the meaning of 'disability' as perceived by people with disabilities themselves. The critiques also argued that increasing dependence on using euphemisms rather than labels to openly communicate about disabilities have come into use wherein denying disability have contributed towards limiting the numerous stigma and thwart prevention efforts.

Overall Analysis of Notions and Models of Disability

Though there has not been much grand theorising about disability, it can be argued that almost all studies of disability have a grand theory underpinning them. Disability being a complex and multi-dimensional phenomenon cannot be easily understood by recourse to the unequivocal messages of the contrasting models or discourses of disability. The dominant discourses of disability (*i.e.,* the Medical and Social models) are characterised by unambiguous modes of expression. Overall analysis of the various approaches to disability brought certain essential issues to the forefront. It highlighted marked changes in paradigms for defining disability from the Individual approach or more specifically the Medical model to the Social approach. Review of differing expressions and manifestations of the Individual approach or the 'Personal tragedy theory' reveals that some of them were predominantly medical or biological while the others were concerned with identity or negotiation of social roles. Hence, they were more concerned with either the physical or psychological concomitants of impairment. As a result of this, they were found to marginalise the collective needs of people with disabilities for enhanced civil rights and removal of disabling barriers. This ushered in the need to incorporate a shift in paradigm to the social approach which was also found to encompass diverse viewpoints within it. Table 1.3 indicates the prime differences in the rationale of both the models of disability.

While some of the social approach theories were found to be more concerned with structural and material conditions, others laid emphasis on culture and representation. This diversity within the broad domain of Social approach is evident in the works of various theorists. For instance, while Finkelstein (1980) emphasised on the need for sociological explanations of disability

Table 1.3: Differences between the Medical and Social Models

Medical Model Thinking	*Social Model Thinking*
Child is faulty	Child is Valued
Diagnosis	Strengths and Needs defined by self and others
Labeling	Identify Barriers and develop solutions
Impairment becomes Focus of attention	Outcome based programme designed
Assessment, monitoring, programmes of therapy imposed	Resources are made available to Ordinary services
Segregation and alternative services	Training for Parents and Professionals
Ordinary needs put on hold	Relationships nurtured
Reentry if normal enough OR Permanent Exclusion	Diversity Welcomed, Child is Included
Society remains unchanged	Society Evolves

Source: Adapted from Micheline Nason, 1994; Rieser, 2000.

to accommodate 'social death' along with 'social barriers', Barnes (1996) maintained that the oppression of people with impairments can be explained with reference to material and cultural forces. Oliver (1990) opined that disability was a resultant of complex interaction of the 'mode of production and the central values of the society concerned'. Similarly, while the modern materialists maintained that capitalism subjected people with disabilities to a specific and explicit form of exclusion and that social inclusion can be achieved only with the replacement of the exclusionary capitalist system, the Systems approach emphasised the need to observe the phenomenon of disability from different systems prevalent in the society as it would enable people to challenge and overcome the compulsory selectivity has been usually used to classify and describe people as objects in a functionally differentiated society. Despite differing perceptions and understanding of disability by various theorists, the social model continues to act as a philosophical base and catalyst for increasing the politicisation or mobilisation of the movement of people with disabilities.

TAX INVOICE

BOOKS

Sold By:

REKHTA FOUNDATION
Gyan Avenue 12 Pragati Market
Ashok Vihar Phase-II, New Delhi
North West Delhi 110052
Delhi
India
State Code : 07
Ph: 9899492060
GSTIN No.: 07AABTR9771N1ZO

Invoice No. : RMP202049455
Invoice Date : 16/03/2024
Order No. : 38598
Order Date : 11/03/2024

Delivered To:

Pittala Devank
H. No 4-4-79, Zaheer pura, guttala bazar, khammam

Khammam 507003
Telangana
India
State Code : 36

Payment Method : cod
Shipped By : Bluedart Surface - Select 500gm
AWB No. : 77939436642
eWaybill No. :

Description	HSN	Qty	Unit Price	Unit Disc.	Taxable Value	IGST	Total
Visual Impairment - Hardcover Model : Hardcover SKU : 43990868590829		1	675.00	0.00	675.00	0	675.00
Shipping Charges					89.00	0.00	89.00
Net Total		1					764.00

Net Amount Payable (In Words):	Seven Hundred And Sixty Four Rupees Only

All disputes are subject to Delhi jurisdiction only. Goods once sold will only be taken back or exchanged as per the store's exchange/return policy.

Authorised Signature for
REKHTA FOUNDATION

Whether tax is payable under reverse charge No

2

Visual Impairment

Disability as a linguistic term is composite comprising of people with a large variety of unrelated characteristics. However, through the processes of separation and practices of defining society's responsibility they have been separated from the rest. It includes diverse categorisation within itself, of which those having visual impairment constitutes focuss of the book.

The Persons with Disabilities (Equal Opportunities, Protection of Rights and Full Participation) Act, 1995 divides the inability to see into two categories of Blindness and Low Vision. According to the Act, 'Person with low vision' means a person with impairment of visual functioning even after treatment or standard refractive correction and who uses or is potentially capable of using vision for the planning or execution of a task with appropriate assistive device'.

NSSO defined visual disability as loss or lack of ability to execute tasks requiring adequate visual acuity. For the survey, visually disabled included— (a) those who did not have any light perception – both eyes taken together, and (b) those who had light perception but could not correctly count fingers of hand (with spectacles/contact lenses if he/she used spectacles/ contact lenses) from a distance of three metres (or 10 feet) in good day light with both eyes open. Night blindness was not considered as visual disability.

Blindness

Blindness comes under the broad category of visual impairment. It can be defined according to the purpose for which vision is required. There can be 'medical blindness', 'legal blindness', 'occupational blindness', and 'educational blindness'. Lowenfeld (1963) referred to blindness as central visual acuity of 20/200 or if there is a field vision in which the peripheral field becomes contracted to such an extent that the widest diametre subtends to an angular distance no greater than 20 degrees. For educational purposes, individuals regarded as blind are so severely impaired that they must be taught to read by Braille or aural methods (Hallahan and Kauffman, 1991).

A person is regarded to be legally blind when his/her best corrected central acuity is less than 20/200 (perfect visual acuity is 20/20) in the better eye, or if the side vision is narrowed to 20 degrees or less in the better eye. It is important to note here that people who are legally blind may still have some useful vision.

In India, according to the Ministry of Human Resource Development, Government of India, the blind are those who suffer from any of the following conditions:

- Total absence of sight; or
- Visual acuity not exceeding 6/60 or 20/200 (Snellen) in the better eye with correcting lenses; or
- Limitation of the field of vision subtending an angle of 20 degrees or worse.

The Effects of Blindness

On the basis of causative factors, people having blindness can be categorised as congenitally blind and adventitiously blind. Congenitally blind refers to those people who have never experienced sight and are unable to visualise visual concepts. Such people have to conceptualise ideas about objects and reality through any other means other than vision. Adventitiously blind are those who have developed blindness later in life. The loss of sight might be gradual or abrupt after experiencing the world through the medium of vision.

The effects of impairment of vision have been found to extend from both perceptual and non-perceptual domains of development resulting in fragmentation of learning in general and academic performance in particular. The unexpressed feeling of loss of sight is frequently associated with helplessness, inferiority, mobility related stress and anxiety, depression, loss of self-efficacy and poor performance (Meighan, 1970; Singh and Akhtar, 1971; Teare, 1985; Bhardwaj, 1995; Jindal-Snape, Kato and Maekawa, 1998; Rosenblum, 2000).

Since the desired outcome of life is preparation for independent living and to become a contributing member of the society, blind individuals are posed with several problems herein. Physical constraints lead to developmental delays in motor skills and physical competence thereby giving rise to feelings of helplessness and dependence. Due to such difficulties, only a few blind people were considered to be successful in attaining full independence and full identity (Rice, 1984). Several researchers held that restricted mobility affects development of identity (Pollock et al, 1997; Howard, 1996). From an interactionist perspective, identity development takes place in different interplay situations with peers (Mead, 1934). For those with restricted mobility, constant presence of adults or other support services can cause individuals to become more dependent. Most researches indicate that blind persons maintain negative or lower self-esteem.

Of the numerous problems experienced by visually challenged individuals, the influence that additional physical effort upon the alteration of feelings emerged as one of the dominant factors. Many regarded effort as a very important source of emotional disturbance and supported their belief with several examples and illustrations. It is held that disturbances occur when one has to abandon his own methods by which he or she can manipulate his or her visual environment conveniently and substitute it by the socially approved procedure of the sighted.

Cutsforth (1951) while investigating schools for the blind to study the effect of over supervision and over-zealousness in training towards visual respectability found that many students were haunted constantly by the feeling that they were being watched and observed. This feeling followed them even in the privacy of their own rooms. (this is in conjunction with Sartre's concept of gaze). Kirk and Gallagher (1986) also reported that individuals with visual handicap were not markedly affected in terms of their intellectual abilities, their perception of other sense was not substantially different from that of the sighted persons, their language development was affected only in those areas where the meaning of words are dependent on visual concepts and their self-esteem and self-confidence were not distorted except when a peer group negatively influenced their attitude.

Low Vision

Low vision is a reduced level of vision that cannot be fully corrected with conventional glasses. It is not the same as blindness. Unlike a person who is blind, a person with low vision has some useful sight. However, low vision usually interferes with the performance of daily activities, such as reading or driving. A person with low vision may not recognise images at a distance or be able to differentiate colors of similar tones. The World Health Organisation defines a person who needs to be assessed for low vision care as someone 'who has impairment of visual functioning even after treatment and/or standard refractive correction, and has a visual acuity of less than 6/18 down to and including light perception, or a visual field of less than 10 degrees from the point of fixation, but who uses, or is potentially able to use, vision for the planning and/ or execution of task.'

Low vision has a significant impact onpeople's lives. People with low vision maystruggle to look after themselves without help. Low vision affects theirstatus in the eyes of others and can make social situations difficult. It reduces theability of people to pursue an education, tolook after their children, and to earnan income. People with low vision are alsoat greater risk of falls and death.

Prevalence and Incidence of Visual Impairment: Indian Scenario Across the country, 45,571 rural and 24,731 urban households were surveyed in rural and urban areas, respectively from 4,637 villages and 3,354 urban blocks. The number of disabled persons enumerated was 49,300 in rural and 26,679 in urban India. According to the survey estimates, the number of disabled persons in the country was 18.49 million during July to December, 2002, and they formed about 1.8 per cent of the total estimated population. A comparative analysis of visual impairment in different rounds of NSSO is given in Table 2.1 indicating the prevalence and incidence of visually disabled persons per 1,00,000 persons for rural and urban areas.

Table 2.1: Prevalence and Incidence of Visually Disabled Persons per 1,00,000 Persons

All-India Sector	*36th round (July – December, 1981)*			*47th round (July – December, 1991)*			*58th round (July – December, 2002)*		
	Male	*Female*	*Persons*	*Male*	*Female*	*Persons*	*Male*	*Female*	*Persons*
(1)	(2)	(3)	(4)	(5)	(6)	(7)	(8)	(9)	(10)
				Prevalence rate					
Rural	444	670	553	471	548	525	276	326	296
Urban	294	425	356	263	346	302	163	228	194
				Incidence rate					
Rural	32	45	38	22	28	25	10	16	13
Urban	23	38	30	15	25	20	7	10	9

Source: NSSO Report, 2002.

Table 2.2 provides details for the country as a whole, indicating that the prevalence of visual disability has decreased marginally between 1981 and 1991, and substantially between 1991 and 2002.

Table 2.2: NSSO Report—Prevalence of Visual Disability

Year	*Rural*	*Urban*	*Total*
1981	–	–	34, 70, 000
1991	33, 35, 000	6, 70, 000	40, 05, 000
2002	22, 57, 500	5, 69, 200	28, 26, 700

Source: NSSO Report, 2002.

Table 2.3: Age Group and Visual Impairment

(*Number of disabled persons per 100,000 persons*)

Age	*Rural*		*Urban*	
Group	*Blindness*	*Low Vision*	*Blindness*	*Low Vision*
0 – 4	32	5	30	5
5 – 9	48	12	73	16
10--14	52	22	82	10
15 –19	56	21	44	13
20 – 24	65	23	56	18
25 – 29	68	17	43	20
30 – 34	77	16	30	19
35 – 39	75	32	53	20
40 – 44	128	43	79	30
45 – 49	183	65	105	39
50 – 54	266	124	182	98
55 – 59	431	234	283	122
60 & above	1733	747	1087	459
ALL	**210**	**86**	**140**	**54**

Source: NSSO Report, 2002.

It is observed from Table 2.3 that the prevalence rate is highest in the age group, 60 years and above for both blindness and low vision. The trend for higher incidence rate for both conditions in rural and urban areas is similar, i.e., 1,733 and 1,087 for blindness and 747 and 459 for low vision. The lowest prevalence is observed in the age group of zero to four years with 32 and 30 cases of blindness and five cases each of low vision among the rural and urban inhabitants. While, there is a steady rise of blindness with an increase in age, it is not so for low vision. However, in the age group of 55 to 59, there is a marked increase in the prevalence of both blindness and low vision in both rural and urban areas. It appears that visual impairment is an old age problem. About 68 to 72 per cent acquired visual impairment at the age of 60 years and above.

The onset of visual impairment seems to start progressing between the ages of 35 and 44 years. In the remaining age-groups (at onset) from 0-4 years, the percentages were found to be quite low –one per cent or less. It is worth noting that both in the rural and urban sectors, the percentages tend to be higher in the first three age-groups (0-4, 5-9 and 10-14 years) than those in the next four age groups. The results suggest that apart from old age, visual impairment tends to manifest during the early years of life, one to two per cent being visually impaired at birth (Table 2.4). The distribution appears to be identical both for the blind and persons with low vision, for rural and urban, and for male and female (Tables 2.5 and 2.6).

Table 2.4: Age at the Onset of Visual Disability

(Per 1,000 distribution of persons 60 years and above with blindness or low vision by age at onset of disability)

Category across the country	*Disability Since birth*	*Age of onset*										
		0-4	*5-9*	*10-14*	*15-19*	*20-24*	*25-29*	*30-34*	*35-44*	*45-59*	*60 & Above*	*Total*
Blindness												
Rural Male	21	5	8	7	4	2	2	10	45	196	699	1000
Rural Female	17	8	10	8	4	6	8	5	26	238	673	1000
Rural Persons	19	7	9	7	4	4	5	7	34	220	684	1000
Urban Male	18	6	6	10	5	4	1	19	23	301	606	1000
Urban Female	9	12	5	9	14	0	1	7	21	288	633	1000
Urban Persons	13	9	5	10	10	2	1	12	22	294	621	1000
All Male	21	5	7	7	4	2	2	12	41	214	683	1000
All Female	15	8	9	8	6	5	7	5	25	246	666	1000
All Persons	18	7	8	8	5	4	5	8	32	233	673	1000
Low Vision												
Rural Male	13	2	6	4	3	2	0	2	6	234	729	1000
Rural Female	2	8	5	3	0	1	2	0	12	259	708	1000
Rural Persons	7	6	5	3	1	2	1	1	9	248	717	1000
Urban Male	12	0	1	4	0	0	1	0	15	231	727	1000
Urban Female	2	2	0	3	0	7	0	0	25	254	709	1000
Urban Persons	5	1	0	3	0	4	1	0	21	245	716	1000
All Male	13	2	5	4	3	2	0	2	7	233	729	1000
All Female	2	7	4	3	0	2	1	0	14	258	708	1000
All Persons	6	5	4	3	1	2	1	1	11	248	717	1000

Source: NSSO Report, 2002.

Tables 2.5 and 2.6 provide figures of blind persons and persons with low vision perthousand in terms of causes of blindness and lowvision as reported by the NSSO report.

Table 2.5: Distribution of Blind Persons per 1,000 by Cause of Blindness Sex-wise and Sector-wise—All India

All-India Cause of Blindness	*Rural*			*Urban*			*Rural + Urban*		
	Male	*Female*	*Person*	*Male*	*Female*	*Person*	*Male*	*Female*	*Person*
(1)	(2)	(3)	(4)	(5)	(6)	(7)	(8)	(9)	(10)
Sore eyes during first month life	5	2	3	2	1	1	4	2	3
Sore eyes after one month	8	4	6	10	7	8	8	5	6
Severe diarrhea before age six	9	5	7	5	11	8	8	6	7
Cataract	187	233	212	214	183	196	192	223	209
Glaucoma	54	51	52	64	93	80	56	59	58
Corneal opacity	26	17	21	24	54	40	25	24	25
Other eye diseases	186	157	170	171	158	164	183	157	169
Small pox	53	42	47	43	31	36	51	40	45
Burns	4	4	4	4	0	2	4	3	3
Injury other than burns	50	28	38	73	26	47	54	28	27
Medical/surgical intervention	21	23	22	48	49	49	26	28	27
Old age	212	281	250	158	234	200	202	272	241
Other reasons	91	54	70	89	62	74	90	55	71
Not unknown	85	94	90	93	86	89	87	92	90
Total	**1000**	**1000**	**1000**	**1000**	**1000**	**1000**	**1000**	**1000**	**1000**

- Total includes not recorded cases of 'cause of blindness'.

Source: NSSO Report, 2002.

Table 2.6: Per 1000 Distribution of Persons with Low Vision by Cause of Low Vision for Each Sex and Sector—All-India

All-India Cause of Low Vision	*Rural*			*Urban*			*Rural + Urban*		
	Male	*Female*	*Person*	*Male*	*Female*	*Person*	*Male*	*Female*	*Person*
(1)	(2)	(3)	(4)	(5)	(6)	(7)	(8)	(9)	(10)
Sore eyes during first month life	1	0	1	0	2	1	1	0	1
Sore eyes after one month	5	0	2	3	5	4	5	1	3
Severe diarrhea before age six	8	2	5	5	9	7	8	3	5
Cataract	272	287	280	293	405	358	276	309	294
Glaucoma	36	29	32	41	38	40	36	31	33
Corneal opacity	59	39	48	22	8	14	53	33	42
Other eye diseases	121	100	109	221	122	163	137	104	119
Small pox	14	7	10	92	34	58	69	29	47
Burns	2	4	3	3	3	3	2	4	3
Injury other than burns	64	28	44	92	34	58	69	29	47
Medical/surgical intervention	21	13	17	23	31	28	22	16	19
Old age	236	342	295	156	228	198	2o23	321	278
Other reasons	38	31	34	65	43	52	42	33	37
Not unknown	111	108	110	58	59	59	102	99	101
Total	**1000**	**1000**	**1000**	**1000**	**1000**	**1000**	**1000**	**1000**	**1000**

- Total includes not recorded cases of 'cause of low vision'.

Source: NSSO Report, 2002.

About 24 per cent of the respondents of the survey reported 'old age' as the major cause since 21 per cent reported of 'cataract'. 'Other eye diseases' was reported to be the cause in about 17 per cent cases. Although a marginal difference was found in gender and rural–urban distribution, the pattern remains same.The pattern of distribution also remains the same for persons with low vision as that for the blind. About 10 per cent were unaware of the probable cause of their low vision and about 57 per cent reported it was due to 'old age' or 'cataract'. The other major causes for low vision were found to be 'other eye diseases' (12 per cent), 'injury other than burns' (five per cent), 'corneal opacity' (four per cent), etc.

3

Policies and Perspectives on the Education of People with Disabilities

The vigour to achieve Education for All (EFA) by 2015 has led to a focuss on the barriers to participation in basic education for marginalised groups (UNESCO, 2010). Lack of sustainability in providing access to basic education by many disabled children and young people now holds focuss. Historically, problems impeding access to education have been seen as being located within an individual disabled person, who was often medically defined by their impairment. In this view, disabled children were and are still perceived as the ones who must adapt in order to be 'integrated' into the mainstream schooling system, or choose to be educated in a separate 'special' education system.

Education of the Disabled: International Scenario

Special or Residential Schools

Within the educational setup, it is generally the fittest and the brightest students who are given preference. These attitudes have their foundations on certain normative role expectations. The normative phenomenon is based on the historical perspective of education as a tool to train a work or task force. This kind of a set-up required physically strong or 'able bodied' individuals with a mental capacity to fulfill certain basic functions. Considering the disabled individuals as deviants from the mainstream educational system, the segregated or special schools were initiated. The Movement for rights of the disabled gathered momentum from 1960s onward based on the Scandinavian concept about normalisation of difference, the US concept of the Least Restrictive Environment and the Warnock Report of 1978 in United Kingdom. These initiatives sensitised the masses and various international agencies about diverse issues of the disabled. Before the emphasis shifted towards the concept of least restrictive environment and inclusive classroom, education of children with visual impairments was often conducted in large residential/special state schools. The chief aim behind these residential schools was to address children with diverse needs as well as to the future education of children with visual impairment. These schools enabled students to receive a curriculum that cannot be provided in the general education classroom. Adaptations both in terms of materials and equipment are necessary to fully utilise the remaining senses of the visually challenged students. According to Frampton and Kerney (1953), residential school for the visually impaired may be defined as: 'A boarding school offering education and care to blind children from ages three to twenty-one, or from pre-school through the high school. Educationally speaking, these schools attempt to provide complete education and care for the blind children. These services include medical, academic, musical, social, vocationalcourses, placement, and follow-up.'

Tutle (1986) also confirms that the oldest, the most comprehensive and the most expensive delivery model is the residential school. It provides basic array of services:

- Instructional services including classroom, educational materials and equipment, offices and storage, teachers, aides and other specialists;
- Food services including fully equipped kitchen, dining room, cooks, and other personnel;

- Residential services including furnished rooms, linen, laundry, house-parents, and other personnel;
- Extracurricular and recreational services, both on the campus and the community;
- Healthcare services including clinic and medical staff; and
- Maintenance and administrative services.

The entire campus of the residential school is designed, equippedand staffed specifically to meet the needs of the visually impaired children. In addition to the classroom teachers, there may beother specialists in physical education, orientation and mobility, activities of daily living, music, craft teaching, occupational therapy, career counselling, vocational counselling, social work and psychology. The educational materials, educational and mobility devices and specialised equipment are accessible to all the students throughout the campus.

Gideon et al (1992) have defined residential school as: '*A school in which the pupils are provided dormitory accommodation and live apart from normal family environment other than holidays and weekends.*' Generally, a residential school avails grant-in-aid from the State Department of Social Welfare or such other department, mobilises public support as donations, endowments, sponsorship of meals or special events. The residential schools are symbols of public charity, pity and compassion for the visually impaired children. Most schools are managed by public charitable organisations and supported by the State Departments of Social Welfare.

According to Lowenfeld (1983), however, the residential school for the blind has undergone a decisive change in character. It now plays a dominant role in channelising the pupils who have become adjusted into the mainstream society. Lowenfeld (1973) had proposed three general principles for adapting instruction to the educational needs of visually impaired students: concrete experiences, unifying experiences and learning by doing. According to Lowenfeld is important that students with visual impairment to acquire an understanding of shape, size, texture, etc., through tactile observation of real objects in natural settings. Besides this they also need to acquire visual experience and unify knowledge. For this, it is essential to develop explore the environment and acquire experiences by systematic stimulation.

The Response to Intervention Model (RTI) is a multi-tiered framework that has been designed to meet the needs of all students. It brings acquired information about each student with evidence-based instructional approaches so that the teachers and related service providers can recognise and respond to the students needs (Brown-Chidsey and Steege, 2005; Fuchs and Fuchs, 2006). Fig 3.3 depicts the RTI model.

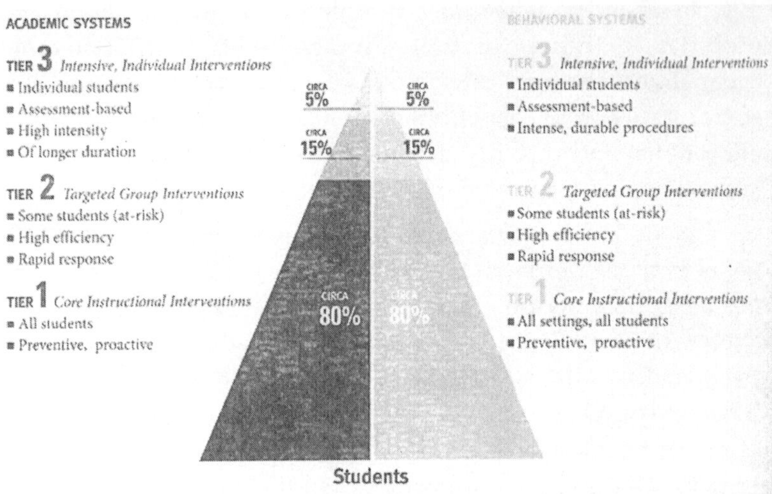

Fig 3.1: RTI Model.

Tier one incorporates universal screening to detect if children need any additional support or enhancement to meet the success and progress monitoring to ensure that the support provided is appropriate for the child. Children with visual impairment would need additional help to prosper in Tier one activities in order to keep pace with their sighted peers. In Tier two, targeted supports and services are provided collaboratively on general and special educational resources, and additional resource personnel if needed. This Tier would include activities which would lay emphasis on individualised or group instruction about independent living skills along training in orientation and mobility.

Tier three would include intensive supports and services to address specific student strengths and weaknesses. For students with visual impairments this Tier would include a separate curriculum, learning of Braille and other means of communication. Adaptations may also needed in curriculum. There would be a core curriculum offering standard lessons in English or language arts, mathematics, social studies, health, etc. Apart from this, the core curriculum can also have an expanded core curriculum including use of assistive technology, orientation and mobility, independent living skills, career education, etc. Training in language skills can be facilitated through the use of optical tools, echo reading along with writing skills through the use of bold-lined paper, mounted magnifiers, etc. Apart from these, the students also taught sex education, recreation and leisure skills.

Recent Trends in Non-integrated or Special Education for Disabled Children in India

Traditionally, most children with special needs in India were being served in the special or residential schools. The residential schools have survived and grown in numbers over the years. At present, 3,000 such schools are there catering to the needs of nearly 1,00,000 children with disabilities. Among them, approximately 900 are institutions for hearing impaired children, 400 for children with visual impairment, 1,000 for mentally retarded and the remaining 700 for children with other types of disabilities (Kundu, 2000). In the rural areas, out of the total 5,86,465 villages in the country, a mere 241 villages have the facilities for special schools. In these villages, there are a total of 272 schools, of which 73 schools have the facility to impart education to the blind, 128 schools to deaf and dumb, 169 schools to orthopedically handicap, 70 schools to mentally retarded and 25 to various other types of disabilities. In these schools, only 9,843 children are reported to be enrolled, of which 1,471 (14.94 per cent) are blind, 3,080 (31.29 per cent) are deaf and dumb, 3,000 (30.48 per cent) are orthopedically handicapped, 1,202 (12.21 per cent) are mentally retarded and 1,090 (11.07 per cent) suffer from other types of handicap. The state governments as well as the Union Government are making more allocations for further expansion of these schools (Sixth All India Educational Survey, 1999).

Residential School Education for Students with Visual Impairment in India

The first school for the visually impaired was founded in India at Amritsar by Miss Annie Sharp in 1887. It was shifted to Dehradun during 1903 and is now called the Sharp Memorial School for the Blind. In the same year, Mr Bihari Shah started the Calcutta School for the Blind. The year 1889 witnessed the establishment of an institution for the visually impaired run by the Canadian Presbyterian Mission established at Indore. Ms A. K. Askwith established the Palayamkottai school for the Blind in 1890. A class for the visually impaired was started at Ranchi by Ms O'Connor in 1893. In 1896, the Canadian Presbyterian Mission started a class for the visually impaired at Ujjain. The Mukti Mission established a Home for the Blind at Kodgaon, Poona in the year 1900. In the same year, Ms Millard founded the American Mission School for the Blind which was subsequently renamed as the Dadar School for the Blind. In 1901, Mr M.M. Srinivas established the School for the Deaf and the Blind at Mysore. The Victoria Memorial School for the Blind established in Mumbai in 1902.

The year 1915 witnessed the foundation of the Mehsana School for the Blind by the Baroda State. In 1917, the N.S.D. Industrial Home for the Blind was established in Mumbai. The foundation for The Blind Relief Association in Mumbai was laid in 1919. This organisation later established centres at Chalisgaon, Valsad and Surat. Mr B.N. Mitter founded the Patna School for the Blind in 1922. In 1925, Happy Home for the Blind was founded in Mumbai. In the same year Mr Sahabzada Aftab Ahmed Khan founded Ahmadi School for the Blind at Aligarh. The Madras Association for the Blind was established in 1929. Dr Kugelberg founded the Tirpattur School for the Blind during the same tenure period. In 1932, the K. K. School and Home for the Blind was founded at Bhavnagar. During 1934, Mr V.H. Telang founded the Poona School and Industrial Home for the Blind. The Government School for the Deaf and the Blind was established at Hyderabad in 1939. Dr Mary Scott started Kalimpong School for the Blind in 1939. The foundation for the All India Lighthouse for the Blind at Calcutta was laid by Mr

Subhodh Chandra Ray in 1941. St Dunstan of London established the St Dunstan's Hostel for Indian War Blinded at Dehradun in 1943 which presently accommodates the National Institute for the Visually Handicapped.

The Blind Relief Association established in New Delhi in 1944. In 1945, the Navrangpura School for the Blind was established at Ahmedabad. The Model School for the Blind established at Dehradun in 1949. Shri Jagdish Patel established the Blind People's Association at Ahmedabad in the year 1950.

In 1951, the National Association for the Blind was established in Mumbai. The Blind Boys Academy was established at Narendrapur, West Bengal in 1957. In 1958, Mrs Rehmut Sultan Fazelbhoy, a trained teacher of the blind and a member of the Executive Council of NAB (I) was successful in admitting three blind boys in New Activity School in Mumbai, of which Mrs Dolat Dungaji was the Principal. Such efforts, however, remained isolated to a few cases in the 1960s and 70s. Thereafter, what started as an experiment in Mumbai gained rapid grounds in a decade's time, and in the years that followed became a movement that spread in the other parts of the country.In the intervening period, NAB, India provided school and college going blind children a variety of support services in the form of scholarships, free distribution of braillers and other assistive devices, voluntary readers' service and so on.

The foundation for the Divine Light School for the Blind at Whitefield, Bangalore was laid in 1958. A School for the Blind was established at Bhubneshwar in 1960. The Andhra Blind Mission School established at Nasrapur in 1962. During 1963, the Bharat Blind School was established at Shahdara, Delhi. The Shree Ramna Maharishi Academy for the Blind was established at Bangalore in 1969.

A large number of schools for the visually impaired were established across the country during 1981 as a part of observation of the International Year of Disabled Persons. The Persons with Disabilities Act, 1995 prepared the ground for the promotion of all modes of education including residential education. The Scheme of Assistance for the Promotion of

Voluntary Education, 1998 also supported the establishment of special schools for visually impaired children with multiple disabilities. During the year 2000, approximately 300 schools for the visually impaired across the country were catering to the needs of 20,000 visually impaired children.

Analysis of the trend of efforts concerning the residential schools makes it evident that the subsequent six decades since the establishment of the first special school for the blind in India at Amritsar in 1887 witnessed the emergence of several special schools in different parts of the country. Although the blind children for the most part stayed in these institutions and received education along with some elementary trades that led them to some kind of vocational rehabilitation, later not much could be achieved through this system of education, in so far as their socio-economic rehabilitation was concerned. Concern about their isolation from mainstream, standard of education and expensive nature of the system occupied a major part of the issues that needed immediate attention. The various backlogs and barriers of the system of education made it imperative to undertake more focussed and comprehensive efforts for deriving optimum benefits. It is within this perspective that the present study aims to look into the diverse factors affecting self-esteem, adjustment pattern and academic performance of blind individuals. This necessitates us to explore the comprehensive literature available on the concerned population.

Integrated Educational Settings: International Scenario

Harping on the context of equalisation of educational opportunities integration was adopted as the central theme of education for the disabled. Although there seems to be lack of adequate consensus regarding its definition, the term 'integration' is used as a collective noun for all attempts to avoid segregated and isolated education of students with disability. Its scope ranges from the actual integration in regular and special schools (or classes) to measures to reduce the outflow of regular education to special education. Hence, for functional purposes, it is referred to, as placing disabled children in a community school with special support services, teachers, books, etc. The Warnock Committee Report (1978) stated that—

> '...Integration for the disabled means a thousand things. It means the absence of segregation. It means able to be treated like everybody else. It means the right to work, to go to cinemas, to enjoy outdoor sports, to have a family life and a social and a love life, contributing materially to the community, to have the usual choices of association, movement and activity, to go on holiday to the usual places, to be educated up to University level with one's non-handicapped peers, to travel without fuss on public transport..., this passage catches the part of changing attitudes to handicap in all its manifestations' (J. Fish, 1981, p. 89).

The present day philosophy is that all disabled people should have the opportunity to obtain an existence as close to normal as possible. In this regard, mention may be made of the educational rights provided to the disabled at the World Conference on Actions and Strategies for Education; Prevention and Integration, Government of Spain with UNESCO (1981, p.6). For instance:

> 'Every disabled person must be able to exercise his fundamental right to have full access to education, training, culture and information'. (Article 1)

> 'Education, training, culture and information programmes must be aimed at integrating disabled persons into the ordinary working and living environment. Such integration must begin as early as possible in the person's life. In order to bring this about, disabled persons must receive appropriate education and training, whatever their personal situation (in institutions, at home in schools etc.for as long as necessary'. (Article 6)

The process of integration for disabled is based on certain rationale. To begin with, when the disabled are not allowed to attend normal schools they may sense themselves to be somehow inferior. Identifying these children as 'special' has not much positive connotation for them when 'special' implies that they must be kept separate from the other children. This increasing dependency would result in social isolation. Apart from this, the need to know has been identified by psychologists. Jean Piaget for example posits that thinking ability develops because of a drive to use what we already know. The Humanistic psychology makes it clear that there is a hierarchy of needs and that a person deprived of basic satisfaction cannot go on to satisfy the higher needs, like curiosity and autonomy. Thus out of the mainstream society, disabled children will have no scope to develop relationships with the 'normal' individuals. In such a condition it will become difficult for them to try out behaviour that are appropriate and productive for himself, thus failing to find viable alternatives to the responses of the able bodied people. It was hence considered that disabled children might acquire age appropriate skills by observing and imitating developmentally advanced peers in the regular classrooms. Through the process of integration an attempt is made to modify the stereotypical notions of the general mass towards disabled people, creating a suitable social setting where they can be regarded as equivalent to others.

Towards a systematic understanding of integrated programmes they can be grouped in to three aspects:

- *Spatial Aspects:* In a situation where special units or special classes are set up in general schools or even where special school and general school are on the same campus, both the disabled and non-disabled children can familiarise with each others behaviour.
- *Social Aspects:* While attending a special class or unit the disabled children have the opportunity to join the non-disabled in several activities. Since young children are more receptive, social mixing will be useful if started at an early age.
- *Functional Aspects*: Having achieved success at special and social integration level; disabled children can attend any regular class and can participate effectively in the normal activities.

The integrated educational programme can be adopted and implemented on the basis of various models. Their application largely varies according to the nature of the society, topography, administrative and educational system, economic resources, etc. Some of the prominent models adopted are the Resource model, Itinerant model, Cooperative model, etc. In the Resource model, disabled children are enrolled in a regular class, while a special teacher is also available. The regular teacher caters to the general educational programmes while the special teacher caters to instruction in special techniques. In the Itinerant model a disabled child is enrolled in a regular class in his home school where his needs are met through the combined efforts of the regular teacher and the visiting itinerant teachers. Under the cooperative plan, disabled children are enrolled in a special room, from where they can go to the regular classroom for a part of the day.

The Conceptual model of special education is based on Reynolds's framework (1960) and the Deno's Cascade model (1970) of special educational services. The Cascade system (the inverted Pyramid model) displays 11 major administration plans in special education; from the most integrated to the most segregated educational setting.

Most Integrated Plans, 1 and 2.

Most Segregated Plans, 9, 10 and 11.

Type I (Exceptional Pupils)

Plan 1: Special education instructional materials and equipment only; enrolled in a regular day class.

Plan 2: Special educational instructional materials and equipments only; enrolled in a regular day class plus special educational tutors enrolled in a regular day class.

Type II (Exceptional Pupils)

Plan 3: Itinerant or school based tutors; enrolled in a regular day class.

Plan 4: Special education resource room and teacher; enrolled in a regular day class.

Plan 5: Part time special day class where enrolled; receives some academic instruction in as regular day school.

Type III (Exceptional Pupils)

Plan 6: Self contained specials day class where enrolled; received no academic instruction in a regular day class.

Plan 7: Combination of regular and special day school; receives no academic instruction in a regular class.

Plan 8: Special day school.

Type IV (Exceptional Pupils)

Plan 9: Special boarding school or residential school facilities.

Plan 10: Hospital instruction.

Plan 11: Homebound instruction.

In the recent years, there has been growing concern to increase level of access and participation for children with special needs within the regular school setup. This was clearly highlighted in the 'World Declaration on Education For All' (WDEFA, 1990) and in the Salamanca Statement (UNESCO, 1994, p.5). The Salamanca Statement laid down that—

> 'Those with special educational needs must have access to regular schools which should accommodate them within child centreed pedagogy capable of meeting their needs. Regular schools with this orientation is the most effective means of combating discriminatory attitude, creating welcoming communities, building an inclusive society and achieving education for all. Moreover, they provide an effective education to the majority of the children and improve the efficiency and ultimately the cost effectiveness of the entire education system'.

Hoben looking into the purpose of educating disabled children in regular education settings observed that the intention should be to make them an integral part of this environment rather than to be simply present in the regular classes. Realising that integration is the result of the mainstreaming, particularly with reference to student interaction, he suggested that interaction with other students should be encouraged.

Recent Trends in Integrated Education for Children with Disabilities in India

Although the scheme of integrated education for the disabled had been adopted in the Western countries in the late nineteenth century, it gained attention in India much later. Efforts have been made for providing services for people with disabilities to be regarded as a part of its social and economic design in a more inclusive fashion than by segregation. Numerous policies have been made by various Commissions, Committees and acts to make integration a reality in India. In 1944, the Sargent Committee Report emphasised upon making provisions for the education of the handicapped. It stated that they were to be sent to special schools only when the nature and extent of the defects made it necessary. The Kothari Commission (1964-66) accepted that 'experimentation with the integrated programme is urgently required and every attempt should be made to bring in as many children into integrated programme as possible' (p.222). The two advantages underlined by the commission are the 'reduction of costs' and promoting mutual understanding between handicapped and non-handicapped children. In 1974, the scheme of Integrated Education of the Disabled Children (IEDC) was launched, which was modified in 1992. The scheme intends to provide educational opportunities for the disabled children in common schools, to facilitate their retention in the school system. It recommended that the children in special schools are to be integrated in common schools once they acquire communication and daily living skills at the functional level.

The National Policy of Education (1986) recommended integrated education for children with locomotor handicaps and other mild disabilities. The Programme of Action, (1992) also stressed upon the inclusion of educational needs of the handicapped children in planning for Universal Elementary Education. It had stated that—'No child whose educational needs can be met in common with others should be placed in special schools. Those who are placed in special schools should be integrated in general schools as soon as they are ready for it' (MHRD, 1986b, p. 18). The Rehabilitation Council of India Act (1992) and The Persons with Disabilities Act (1995) also emphasised upon the need to ensure that every disabled child has access to free education in an appropriate environment.

Integrated education in India emerged out of compulsion to some extent rather than as an option of a cohesive school system. In 1887, Amy Strap, a missionary from England started the first school for the blind in Amritsar. The objective initially was to provide shelter to destitute girls. The year 1947 witnessed the emergence of quite a number of schools and institutions for the blind, slightly more than thirty. However, education in these institutions was confined only to the primary level and in most cases the students were not admitted before the age of seven. It was only after independence that any major change was brought about in the educational scenario.

In the process of bringing special needs of children under the umbrella of educational services, integration came out as a cost-effective approach and, therefore, the general education system started acceptingspecial needs children in general schools. Integration of such children has been reinforcing better educational practices in general schools. Of the total 8,22,486 schools in the country only 16,294 (2.0 per cent) schools have the integrated education programme. Of these, 11,412 (70.0 per cent) are in rural areas and 4,882 (30.0 per cent) are in urban areas. Further, only 8,782 (53.9 per cent) primary schools, 4,209 (25.8 per cent) upper primary schools and 3,303 secondary and higher secondary schools have integrated educational programme. At present, under the Centrallysponsored scheme of integrated education which was started in 1974, and since then is being implemented in various states, more than 50,000 children with disabilities are reported to benefit by this approach through 15,000 general schools.

Integrated Education for Students with Visual Impairment in India

It was only after independence that any major change was brought about in the educational scenario of blind children among education professionals, voluntary agency administrators and government officials. The period saw the emergence of numerous schools and institutions roughly around two hundred.

Educational professionals concentrated on providing blind children with knowledge at par with their sighted peers. The blind students also received the permission to appear for public examinations.

Efforts were also made in educating blind students in rural areas, when a new avenue of education was explored and implemented at Visnagar, Mehsana District, Gujarat in 1982, i.e., the itinerant teacher facility to cater to the needs of such children. Similar programmes were also implemented at various areas in Haryana, Karnataka and Tamil Nadu supported by various organisations like the Royal Commonwealth Society for the Blind (RSCB), National Association for the Blind (NAB), etc.

At present under the Centrally sponsored scheme of integrated education, children with visual impairment are approximately 8,600 (Sixth All India Educational Survey, 1999). Although education of children with visual impairment is emphasised upon, yet the present service delivery systems have not even covered five per cent of the clientele. There still seems to be a long way to go, in order to in realise education for all children with visual impairment.

Debate between Non-integrated or Special and Integrated Educational Schools

Historically, arguments for placing disabled children in separate or non-integrated schools and homogeneous groups have included four basic points. *Firstly*, the advocates of this placement hold that there is the need to protect students from the painful and harmful experience of repeated failure. *Secondly*, there is the belief that such failure results in permanent and irrevocable damage. They hold that from the humanitarian point of view, it ensures protection from frustration and feelings of inferiority derived from undue competition (Quay, 1963). *Thirdly*, the advocates hold that there is the need to target slower, more direct instructional methods in both academic and behavioural skills to children requiring special assistance (Brown, 1974; Meyen and Lehr, 1980). Special schools according to them can provide them with a secure educational setting where controlled and adaptable environment with specialised equipment provides opportunities for simulation of natural environment, reduction of distractions and intensive individualised instruction. *Finally*, there is the concern that children left in the regular setting would fall further and become stigmatised by their peers. Through such arguments, the advocates of special schools for the disabled indicate that merely leaving children in the regular school environment alone does not ensure integration and may seriously harm their academic and social development. Hatlen (1989) taking up the case of blind children held that although the students attended their neighbourhood school they were not integrated. Laird (1992) also maintained that some of the blind students were not integrated completely in regular schools and became uninvolved spectator, 'isolated islands in the mainstream' (p. 213).

The supporters of integration of disabled children maintain that separating children overtly stigmatises them, condemns them permanently to the bottom track. They regard this system as a form of social control. Bilken (1989) perceived it as a method adopted by the society to remove disabled children from the mainstream and saw special education as a 'safety valve' for students who were unable to succeed in the regular class. The separate system of education leads to segregation and labelling of children excluding them from the activities of the mainstream society. The disabled child in such circumstances has no opportunity to develop relationship with anyone except, others with disabilities and the adults who affect his or her life. Thus, the children fail to try out behaviour, which are most appropriate and productive for them. Moreover, if disabled children are not allowed to attend regular schools except with other disabled children, then they may infer themselves to be somehow inferior. The supporters of integration further hold that placing disabled children in special settings lowers others' (parents, teachers, etc) expectations for them. Therefore, according to them, the act of separation deprives contact and is so painful that it counteracts any possible gains (Johnson, 1962; Dunn, 1968; Glass and Smith, 1977). In relation to the problems put forth by the separate system of education, Reynolds (1962) held that the prevailing view is that 'normal' home and school should be preserved if at all possible. When a special placement is necessary to provide suitable care or education, it should be no more special than necessary... Children should be placed in programmes no more of special character than absolutely necessary. There should be continuing assessment of children in special programmes with a view toward returning to more ordinary environment as soon as possible.' On the economic front, it was held that this system proves to be cost generating both in terms of manpower as well as capital.

Inclusive Education: Quality Education for All

The principle of inclusive education was first internationally recognised and endorsed in 1994 at the World Conference on Special Needs Education in Salamanca, Spain. Addressing the diverse needs of all students the Salamanca Declaration encouraged governments to design education systems to promote their accessibility in regular schools with a child-centered pedagogy. However, it was the UN Convention on the Rights of Persons with Disabilities (CRPD) in 2006 that established inclusive education as a mechanism to deliver the right to education for people with disabilities. The CRPD in its Article 24 accentuated the need for governments to ensure equal access to an 'inclusive education system at all levels' and provide reasonable accommodation and individual support services to persons with disabilities to facilitate their education. Ratification of the CRPD made the countries legally obliged to provide inclusive quality and free primary and secondary education to all children. As of September 2013, 133 countries and the European Union had ratified the CRPD, with another 23 having signed but not yet ratified.

Inclusive Education for the Disabled: The Indian Scenario

The Government of India, in conjunction with the World Bank, created the Sarva Shiksha Abhiyan (SSA), an initiative which translates to 'Education for All.' It is important to note that although SSA is not a disability-specific programme, but is rather a disability-inclusive programme, with specific aspects that benefit people with disabilities. The programme aims to benefit people with disabilities in numerous ways. *Firstly*, it encompasses a Rs 1,200 allocation per annum for per child with a disability catering to his/her such as expenses towards assistive devices, materials in alternative learning formats etc. to facilitate inclusion into a mainstream classroom. The *second* part of SSA has specified that each district will formulate its own plan for children with disabilities, while the *final* part mentioned that key institutions will be encouraged to collaborate to further support these students with disabilities thus ensuring their inclusion.

The year 2005 witnessed the drafting of the Action Plan for Inclusion in Education of Children and Youth with Disabilities (IECYD) by the Ministry of Human Resource Development.The plan envisioned that all children with a disability will have access to mainstream education; in order to facilitate this, the government, specifically collaborating between the Rehabilitation Council and the National Council for Teacher's Education, will ensure that there are adequate numbers of teachers trained in inclusive education as well as the proper physical and ideological infrastructure to facilitate inclusion in schools. The plan specifically looks to move from integration towards inclusion, stating, whereas under the Scheme of Integrated Education for the Disabled Children (IEDC) as it stands at present, children with disabilities are placed in a regular school without making any changes in the school to accommodate and support diverse needs, the revised IECYD will, in contrast, modify the existing physical infrastructures and teaching methodologies to meet the needs of all children, including Children with Special Needs. A unique aspect of this plan is that it steps outside the Indian constitution and includesstudents with disabilities outside of the 6-14 age range. Through Integrated Child Development Services (ICDS), anganwadi workers will be trained to identify children with disabilities at an early age, so they can receive early intervention services. While the crucial importance of early intervention cannot be overlooked, the IECYD also discusses accommodations for students with a disability in universities, including a mandatory 'disability coordinator' who provides inclusion services for students with disabilities.

In 2008, the government reformed the Scheme of Integrated Education for DisabledChildren (IEDC) and created the Inclusive Education of the Disabled at the Secondary Stage (IEDSS) which went into effect on April 1st, 2009. IEDC was reformed to take into account the resources provided for students with disabilities aged 6-14 under Sarva Shiksha Abhiyan. The objective of IEDSS is to enable the disabled children who have completed eight years of elementary education to continue their education at the secondary stage in an inclusive environment in regular schools. IEDSS provides students with disabilities age 14-18, studying in public or government-funded schools, Rs 3,000 per school year from the central government to purchase the necessary materials to use to ensure inclusion of the student in the mainstream school system. This can be regarded as the first policy that specifically acknowledges the importance of secondary education for persons with disabilities.

The most recent policy specifically concerning education and people with disabilities isthe Ministry of Social Justice and Empowerment's National Policy for People with Disabilities. Despite the policy being created in 2006, after the 2005 Action Plan, and thetwo policies were created under separate ministries, they are very similar in both the ideologiesthat they were founded on, as well as the actual changes they are trying to make to thesystem. The National Policy for People with Disabilities utilises Sarva Shiksha Abhiyan (in English, Education for All), also created by the Ministry of Social Justice and Empowerment, astheir main mode of implementation of the policy.This policy echoes the 2005 plan of action (made official in 2009) bill by changing special schools in resource centres for peoplewith disabilities and teachers. In addition, the policy seeks to bridge the gap between rural andurban areas by creating more District Disability and Rehabilitation Centres (DDRCs), whichdisseminate information in terms of availability of aids and appliances, ensure themandated three per cent coverage of persons with disabilities in poverty reduction programs andtarget girls with disabilities.

It becomes imperative to note that although policies in India have always leaned towards inclusion these policies often are notperfectly inclusive. Many of them tend to discriminate against people with 'severe' disabilities, or people with intellectual disabilities, especially in terms of mainstream versus special schooling.

An overview of numerous developments and trends in education of people with disabilities in light of different perspectives and approaches, policy perspectives, educational practices and problems have brought certain issues to the forefront. It is obvious that there has been marked shift in paradigms with regard to different educational policies and programmes for optimising the development of people with disabilities by way of special education and ensuring their incorporation into the mainstream society.

4

Barriers in the Education of People with Disabilities

Barriers in the Education of Students with Disabilities in India

Even though several educational policies from the Kothari Commission (1966), NPE (1986) to the Programme of Action (1992) and Persons with Disabilities Act (1995) have laid down certain guidelines for education of children with disabilities within their policy framework, they failed to adequately address some of their basic concerns such as the issues of accessibility, education and employment (Nagarajan, 2001; A Reporter, 2000; Veedon, 1999). In regard to this, mention can be made of the Projected Integrated Education for the Disabled (PIED) which has been subjected to a series of criticism. It is maintained that the expectations were not adequately met. The critiques of PIED hold that the scheme suffered from certain limitations such as there was lack of appropriate assessment tools due to which the categorisation and selection of students was often reported to be arbitrary and incorrect. Due to this, it was centrally focussed on children with mild to moderate disabilities who are not identified while entering school and form substantial portion of the dropouts. As a result of this, the issue of pre-school support was also not adequately addressed (Karnath and Kaur, 1993). The magnitude of the problem was accounted for confinement of the scheme to limited categories of disability (Jangira, 1995). Lack of clarity on the status of special education teachers also resulted in confusion and professional competition (Seetharam, 1982), thereby diluting the purpose of various programmes. Moreover, there was also lack of specific prescribed curriculum and inadequate short-term orientation courses for providing sustained on-going support to classroom teachers (Seetharam, 1982; Nathan, 1991). Due to some of these factors, the approach failed to attain materialisation.

One of the major hurdles limiting the adoption of adequate initiatives to address the needs of the disabled population in India is the unavailability of accurate data on the status of disability in the country. A comprehensive Census survey of mentally and physically challenged people released on August 9, 2004 revealed that there were 21,906,769 disabled people in India in January 2001. Of the total number, 16,388,382 belong to rural communities and 5,518,387 to urban areas. The distribution in terms of sex stands at 12,605,635 males and 9,301,134 females. Of the more than two crore figure visually impaired people account for 48.5 per cent, physically challenged 27.9 per cent, mentally challenged 10.3 per cent, speech impaired 7.5 per cent and hearing impaired 5.8 per cent. According to the Census 2001, there are 2.19 crore people with disabilities in India who constitute 2.13 per cent of the total population. This includes persons with visual, hearing, speech, locomotor and mental disabilities. Seventy five per cent of persons with disabilities live in rural areas, 49 per cent of disabled population is literate and only 34 per cent are employed.

It is evident from Fig 4.1 that the number of disabled people as revealed in the 2001 census is marginally higher than the estimate of the National Sample Survey Organisation (NSSO) of 1.8 crore. Fig 4.2 beneath gives a picture of the disability-wise Segregation of Estimated Population as provided by the National Sample Survey Organisation (NSSO).

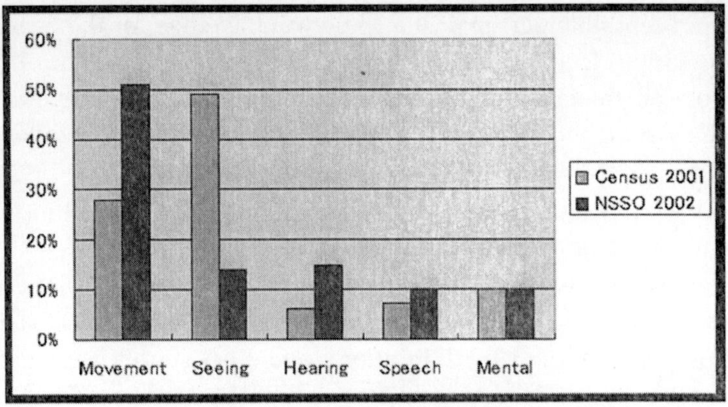

Census 2001 v/s NSSO 2002

Fig 4.1: Number of Disabled People in India.

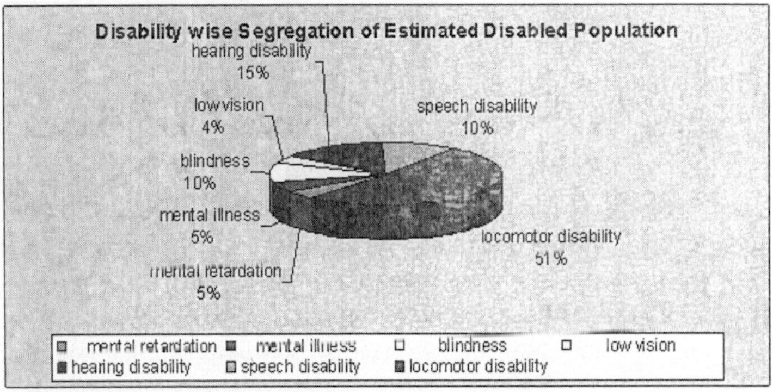

Source: National Sample Survey Organisation, 2002.

Fig 4.2: Disability-wise Segregation of Estimated Population.

Despite various attempts to ensure integration of people with disabilities into the mainstream there is a dichotomy between intent and practice whereby although emphasis is being continuously laid by governments on integration they are also accompanied by segregation policy at the parallel level. Based on NSS data, the World Bank (2007: 64) report categorically states that, 'it is very clear that both educational attainment of all PWD and current attendance of CWD are very poor and far below national averages'. Data suggests that people with disabilities have much lower educational attainment rates, with

52 per cent illiteracy against a 35 per cent average for the general population. It is important to note that illiteracy levels are high across all categories of disability, and extremely so for children with visual, multiple and mental disabilities (and for children with severe disabilities across all the categories).

Apart from the inconsistencies in estimates regarding the total population of people with disabilities in India, there are large discrepancies in the number of CWD identified between census data, school based records through DISE (District Information System for Education), and PAB survey aggregates used by the SSA. According to estimates made under SSA, around 1.5 per cent of children in the 6-14 age groups have special needs, while the 2001 Census data indicates the proportion to be around 2.2 per cent. The picture is more confusing when examined across the states where differences between identification rates are much higher. While some of these discrepancies could be attributed to different definitions, perceptions and indeed training of the enumerators, they certainly raise concerns about the effectiveness and reliability of the identification procedures.

Moreover, although the issue of identification of CWSN has been of main focuss in SSA and the reports note a steady increase in their numbers (See Table 4.1) suggesting that there is growing awareness of the concerns of CWSN, assumptions underpinning the process of identification and assessment need to be critically examined. There are large discrepancies in the number of CWD identified between census data, school based records through DISE (District Information System for Education), and PAB survey aggregates used by the SSA According to estimates made under SSA, around 1.5 per cent of children in the 6-14 age groups have special needs, while the 2001 Census data indicates the proportion to be around 2.2 per cent. Differences in the identification rates are much higher when examined across the states which further aggravate the issue. It becomes evident from data gathered for PAB 2005-06 that while only 0.31 per cent and 0.7 per cent children have been identified with special needs in Rajasthan and Uttar Pradesh, the rates for Maharashtra and Himachal Pradesh were found to be much higher at 2.45 and 2.3 per cent respectively (figures quoted in World Bank, 2007).

Table 4.1: Identification of CWSN

Year	*Total numbers identified as CWSN*
2002-03	6,83,554
2003-04	14,59,692
2004-05	15,92,722
2005-06	20,17,404
2006-07	23,99,905
2007-08	26,21,077

Source: Sarva Shiksha Abhiyan (2007).

Moreover, the SSA documentation does not provide a definition of CWSN other than assuming that this group is synonymous with children with disabilities and all disabilities give rise to need for special education. The SSA in its category titled 'Special Focus Groups Under SSA' does not acknowledge the presence of intersectionalities between the various groupings and how they need to be addressed.

Apart from the unreliability of data on the educational participation of children with disabilities in terms of estimates in the school going age group, much discrepancy also exits in the numbers actually attending school. In a countrywide survey on the enrolment of disabled children in educational institutions in India, the National Centre for Promotion of Employment for Disabled People (NCPEDP) reveal that only a fraction of the disabled get admission into schools and colleges. The survey conducted in 119 universities report an enrolment of only 1,635 students and only 679 to 96 colleges. Further the survey also revealed greater bias towards disabled in schools than colleges. Estimates indicate that only 382 students with disabilities were enrolled in 89 schools while 18 of them cited the existence of special schools to be the reason for not integrating them to regular schools. Mukhopadhyay and Mani (2002) in a NCERT survey, suggested that about 84,000 children with disabilities were enrolled in schools in 1998; and unpublished data gathered for the MHRD suggested that approximately 55,000 children with disabilities were enrolled in schools in 1999. In addition to this despite 'the Office of the Chief Commissioner of Persons with Disabilities stating that not more than four per cent of children with disabilities have access to education', the MHRD claimed in 2004 that 1.08 million children with disabilities were being educated, and by using a very low estimate of the total number of children with disabilities, thus arriving at an estimate of 67.5 per cent of children with disabilities receiving education (MHRD, 2004).

Data on children with disabilities in elementary classes collected under DISE reveals that their number varies from year to year. In the year 2003-04, there were 1.75 million such children as against 1.40 million in 2004-05. However, their number has always remained around one per cent of the total enrolment in elementary classes. In 2006-07, about 1.42 million children with disabilities were enrolled in elementary classes across the country, of which 1.04 million were in primary and 0.38 million in upper primary classes. The percentage of children with disability, in primary, is 0.79 and in upper primary 0.80 of the total enrolment in these classes. The corresponding percentage at the elementary level is 0.80.

Table 4.2: Enrolment According to the Type of Disability

Disability	*Grades*		
	I-V	*VI-VIII*	*IX-X*
Seeing	20.79	32.87	24.02
Hearing	11.69	11.04	11.52
Speech	13.04	8.28	11.77
Moving	27.28	32.09	28.56
Mentally Retarded	19.68	8.62	16.73
Others	7.51	7.10	7.40
% to total enrollment	0.79	0.80	0.80

Source: Compiled from DISE 2006-2007.

Table 4.2 indicates the differences in enrolment according to the type of disability. Almost one in every three children with disabilities in elementary classes has some problem in moving (28.56 per cent). About 24 per cent are visually handicapped6, 12 per cent hard-of-hearing, 12 per cent disabled in speech, about 17 per cent are mentally retarded and seven per cent have other types of disabilities. There are some interesting differences evident as children make the transition from primary to upper primary classes. Compared to 20.79 per cent of children with visual impairment in primary classes, their percentage in upper primary classes is as high as 32.87. On the other hand, figures for children with mental retardation show a significant decline in numbers.

Another area of inequity between persons with disabilities is gender. The Government of India National Census pointed out the extreme inequities between girls and boys with a disability. In number, there are fewer girls than boys with a disability. The hierarchy of Indian society results in selective abortion, female infanticide and female feticide of female children with a disability. A dismal picture for women with disabilities exists in the field of education. In a country like India where the education of girls in general is perceived as liability, the disability further limits their opportunities. In a society where women with disabilities are viewed as a social stigma and objects to be hidden from public view, most of the girls are denied access to education. The most formidable barrier to educational equity for girls with disabilities is their invisibility. The prejudice surrounding their ability and value continues to perpetuate the view that educating them is futile. Only a small proportion of girls with disabilities have access to opportunities of receiving education or attending training courses. Besides this, dearth of programmes and policies explicitly addressing the educational needs of girls with disabilities and failure on the part of gender equity and disability equity programmes to serve their needs further add on their disadvantage. It is imperative to note that although there are policies and programmes addressing education for girls without disabilities it is miserable that despite the needs and associated problems being similar in nature, girls who are disabled are seldom included. Similarly, while strong disability-rights legislation over the years produced a range of efforts to promote educational equity for children who are disabled, few are gender-specific and few include gender-specific components to address the unique barriers facing girls with disabilities.

Apart from aspect of gender and disability, the access to education by girls with disabilities is also affected by their type of disability, the socio-economic status of their family, their race and ethnicity, their area of residence whether urban or rural area and a host of other factors. The incessant relationship between poverty and disability often acts as a significant hurdle. Poverty causes disability, particularly in women and girls and in the face of limited resources, they are more likely than their male counterparts to be deprived of basic necessities such as food and medicine. Hence, disability, in turn, contributes to poverty because of the additional expenses that it can entail. Therefore, girls who are disabled are more likely than their nondisabled peers to grow up in poor families and be placed at an educational disadvantage. In impoverished families, the limited resources available will be used to educate the boys, with the expectation that they will ultimately help support the family. Girls are not likely to be educated, particularly girls who are disabled and need costly disability-related equipment or special transportation. This is more for women with disabilities in rural areas than those living in cities.

Distance to school constitutes an educational barrier for many girls, partly because of safety and cultural prohibitions against females traveling unescorted. For girls with disabilities, such barriers are intensified. The architectural inaccessibility of school buildings (including stairs, narrow corridors, inaccessible desks and equipment, inaccessible bathrooms) is often a major barrier for girls with disabilities.

Although numerous arguments about learning taking place in an 'appropriate' environment, there is lack of critical reflection on the nature of this appropriate environment and about who decides where the child needs to be placed. There is lack of adequate community sensitisation towards the disabled. The efforts of the government in providing educational facilities remain minimal. Moreover, mandatory changes made in the educational systems and services do not suffice to adequately cater to the needs of people with disabilities. More recently, there have been growing concerns regarding the type of school attended by children with disabilities and implications for their integration into society. DISE data does not provide information regarding enrolment figures in special schools. The NSS reveals that in urban areas around 11 per cent of those with disabilities in the five to 18 years age group were enrolled in special schools, while this was less than one per cent in rural areas. This reflects the recent growth in the number of special schools, especially in urban areas. However, these special schools have certain disadvantages which became evident as the number of these schools increased. These institutions reached out to a very limited number of children, largely urban and they were not cost effective. But most important of all, these special schools segregated CWSN from the mainstream, thus developing a specific disability culture. (Janshala, 2003: 1).

Even today separateness is confined not only within the purview of segregated classes but also in 'separate standards' used to evaluate the attainments of these students. Efforts at integrating children with disabilities into mainstream schools have been even less successful. Although the IEDC scheme provides for a wide range of incentives and interventions for the education of children with disabilities including preschool training, counselling for parents, allowances for books and stationery, uniforms, transport, readers and escorts, hostel facilities, other assistive devices, one special teacher for every eight children with disabilities, community involvement, and a resource room in a cluster of eight to 10 schools much is left to be attained. Apart from these, a number of voluntary organisations are also making attempts towards implementing the scheme in the various States. Tables 4.3 and 4.4 give a piecemeal view of the number of students with various forms of disabilities enrolled under the integrated educational programme.

Although numerous recommendations have been made by various policies to ensure adequate infrastructural facilities are the existing situation is one of great dismal. Though it was envisaged that infrastructure in urban and rural areas would be made barrier-free through appropriate schemes and programmes, very few buildings, transportation services, and other public facilities are accessible at present. The PWD Act detailed out the

Table 4.3: Enrollment of Disabled Children in Schools under the Integrated Educational Programme (Stage: Primary)

Area	*Management*	*Type of Disability*					
		Visual	*Hearing*	*Ortho-paedic*	*Mentally Retardation*	*Others*	*Total*
Rural	Govt	1,539	1,307	15,168	1,066	2,070	21,150
	Non-Govt	391	354	2,189	188	80	3,202
	Total	1,930	1,661	17,357	1,254	1,250	24,352
Urban	Govt	896	1,420	5,072	1,694	1,382	10,464
	Non-Govt	982	1,877	3,959	800	1,538	9,156
	Total	1,878	3,297	9,031	2,494	2,920	19,620
Total	Govt	2,435	2,727	20,240	2,760	3,452	31,614
	Non-Govt	1,373	2,231	6,148	988	1,618	12,358
	Total	3,808	4,958	26,388	3,748	5,070	43,972

Source: NCERT, 1998.

Note: Govt includes the Central Government and the State Governments as also Local Bodies and Non-Govt includes Pvt Aided and Pvt Unaided.

Table 4.4: Enrollment of Disabled Children in Schools under the Integrated Educational Programme (Stage: Upper Primary)

Area	*Management*	*Type of Disability*					
		Visual	*Hearing*	*Ortho-paedic*	*Mentally Retardation*	*Others*	*Total*
Rural	Govt	996	533	6,734	369	926	9,558
	Non-Govt	262	264	1,582	67	141	2,316
	Total	1,258	797	8,316	436	1,067	11,874
Urban	Govt	604	904	3,781	271	251	5,811
	Non-Govt	736	581	2,293	572	1,467	5,649
	Total	1,340	1,485	6,074	843	1,718	11,460
Total	Govt	1,600	1,437	10,515	640	1,177	15,369
	Non-Govt	998	845	3,875	639	1,608	7,965
	Total	2,598	2,282	14,390	1,279	2,785	23,334

Source: NCERT, 1998.

Note: Govt includes the Central Government and the State Governments as also Local Bodies and Non-Govt includes Pvt Aided and Pvt Unaided.

architectural and instructional barriers and specified the need for each institute to identify the type of infrastructure that must be modified. Despite the Act laying down detailed guidelines for creating barrier free environment specifying the modifications required regarding corridors, stairways, entrances, lightning or classroom arrangements so as to increase the level of accessibility, most of the schools still did not possess many of the prescribed infrastructural standards. School buildings are predominantly not accessible to people with disabilities; only 18 per cent of SSA schools were 'barrier free,' and the numbers were even lower in some states, with two per cent in Jammu and Kashmir, and six per cent in Bihar. Most of the schools accommodating visually challenged students have to cope with broad stairways with the maximum number of risers and inadequate handrails as they do not have ramps for such special needs. In addition to the classrooms, the location of the toilets, laboratories or cafeteria at a distance requires students to travel across floors. All these factors restrict the mobility of the students with disabilities, thus heightening their dependence on others.

Despite numerous attempts towards integration, the requirements of 'basics' of curricular aspects of such children such as facilities for reading, writing, field trips, standards of attendance, participation, etc., failed to acquire adequate attention and implementation. In a recent attempt by the government to evaluate the curricular issues in CBSE schools it was observed that not only there were difficulties related to the provision of barrier-free environment for such children but also lack of adequate and appropriate study materials such as rarity in availability of Braille books, necessary support services as well as adequate transport services. There are two main types of curriculum in India: plus curriculum, specifically designed for children with disabilities, to increase accessibility (e.g., Braille, large print, reading aids, language/communication for deaf children, communication for children with cerebral palsy), and general curriculum. It is necessary to adapt the general curriculum to the different formats that the plus curriculum is available so as to make it more accessible for children with disabilities.

In both, DPEP and SSA considerable attention has been given to the provision of aids and appliances. The SSA (2003) provides a one-page 'List of aids and appliances required by children with special needs' for four impairment types—visual, hearing, orthopaedic and intellectual. These aids and appliances are largely directed towards equipping the child's functioning (day-to-day and educational), through the provision of aids such as white cane, hearing aid and thick pens. This document also notes the provision of 500 rupees to teachers to develop low cost teaching and learning materials to meet the educational needs of a CWSN in a regular classroom. SSA (2007) notes the increased distribution of aids and appliances to children with CWSN (see Table 4.5). The main focuss however remains on the distribution of wheel chairs, crutches, braces, etc.

Table 4.5: Distribution of Aids and Appliances

Year	*Distribution of aids and appliances to CWSN*
2003-04	121,467
2004-05	286,922
2005-06	370,397
2006-07	711,971
2007-08	832,828

Source: Sarva Shiksha Abhiyan (2007).

While provision of these is indeed very useful and enhances the functional capacity of many children, again these statistics give an incomplete picture. Various problems were found to be associated ranging from difficulty in accessing the provisions, as rehabilitative services tend to be concentrated in urban areas, and the devices given were inappropriate, difficult to repair and maintain in rural areas. Although the SSA specified provision of a Rs 1,200 allocation per annum for per child with a disability catering to his/her such as expenses towards assistive devices, materials in alternative learning formats etc. the major hurdle lies in the issue that the money is funneled through the district or school level, and it is therefore impossible to ensure that it will be spent on the child with a disability. Moreover, under SSA, assistive devices are technically a 'right' and can be obtained outside of the R1200 allocation. However, in reality, SSA often provides these devices through collaboration with outside programmes, and many of these outside programmes have their own restrictions on how often a child with a disability can obtain assistive devices, making these devices a privilege, rather than a right. It is rather sad that despite the stated importance of this population, less than one per cent of the total money allocated for SSA is being used for purposes of inclusion.

Majority of the school personnel are not adequately trained to design and implement educational programmes for students with disabilities in schools. Since the RCI Act of 1992, which set standards for teacher training, there has been shortage of trained teachers and personnel in schools. Although the SSA envisages that training of the teachers analysis of the content merely covers issues of identification and management. Even the numbers of teacher courses are low. As of 2005 less than 0.2 per cent of all SSA teachers had been through this larger programme (quoted in World Bank, 2007), raising concerns about the effectiveness of such programmes impacting pedagogical practices. There is lack of evidence-based practices and even when they are there practitioners/teachers, for various reasons, do not always end up using them. Two major barriers to the implementation of evidence-based practices are the lack of time and inadequate support from administrators. Other barriers include 'pressures associated with high-stakes testing, insufficient materials, a mismatch between teacher style and the practice, a lack of fit between the practice and other methods mandated by the school district, and teachers' lack of in-depth understanding of the practice or forgetting. Practitioners/teachers need incentives and technical assistance in using evidence-based practices, yet little is done to help them learn to apply research to practice.

A nationwide survey by the National Council for Educational Research and Training (NCERT) published in April 2014 which interviewed 203 teachers and 273 students has found that 99 per cent of mentally-challenged children and those with learning disabilities want to study in a regular school. However, 16 states including Maharashtra do not include training for teachers regarding being sensitive to the needs of the syllabus in the syllabus of the Diploma in Education or Bachelor's in Education courses. Despite the Right o Education specifying that children with learning disabilities should study in mainstream schools it was revealed in the study that while 44.5 per cent of the students expressed the need for special attention from teachers, 57.1 per cent teachers have not been trained to meet their needs.

Moreover, government's conceptualisation of the problem remains ingrained with the belief that education and management of disabled children relies on voluntary organisations. Though a number of special schools for blind, deaf, cerebral palsied, mentally handicapped and slow learners are maintained by NGOs there are limitations to their functioning. Their functioning is limited only to the micro level, whereby the geographical logistics of the subcontinent, coupled with the expenditure act as barriers to frequent contact between the NGO groups hence resulting in fragmented and piecemeal services. This largely blurs the intention and efforts made towards mainstreaming. Moreover, much of the efforts are carried out at the micro level and the initiatives taken by the governments and voluntary agencies suffer from lack of continuous funding and good infrastructural support. Besides these, the changing governmental policies further limit the functioning of various agencies. Hence it is imperative to depoliticise the field of special education by establishing a network of collaboration among the various bodies, governmental policy, administrators, professionals, community, parents, etc.

Barriers in the Education of Students with Visual Impairment in India

Although emphasis is continually laid on integrating students with visual impairment into the regular schools, the population/ number of students enrolled in each of the schools surveyed was miniscule. Several reasons emerged on inquiring about the enrolment rates of students with some of the concerned authorities of various institutions aiming to integrate them in mainstream schools. Some of the authorities mentioned that the central problem lay in the attitude of the parents of the children, where some of the parents opined that their children would be best taken care of in special schools with special assistance. They felt that apart from the benefits of special aids and teachers, the issue of being placed with other students having similar needs would be an added advantage and would have a positive impact on the psychological makeup of their children. Moreover, the notion that their children may be subjected to unnecessary criticism, abuse, and unavailability of adequate and essential facilities accounted for some of the apprehensions that seem to restrain the parents from admitting their children to regular schools. Although numerous recommendations have been made to ensure adequate infrastructural facilities are provided for PWD, the existing situation is one of underachievement. Though it was envisaged that infrastructure in urban and rural areas would be made barrier-free through appropriate schemes and programmes, very few buildings, transportation services, and other public facilities are accessible at present. Moreover, much is left to be attained despite the fact that many policies have envisaged the need to adopt adequate measures for creating a barrier-free environments and prescribed guidelines and space standards in the process. Certain issues emerged while observing the schools selected for the study based on the School Observation Checklist, which was prepared in consultation with some concerned authorities as in the light of the standards prescribed by the Integrated Education for the Disabled Act and the PWD Act in 1995.

The PWD Act detailed out the architectural and instructional barriers and specified the need for each institute to identify the type of infrastructure that must be modified, so that the Government can provide financial assistance for such upgrades or modifications. The Act also laid down detailed guidelines for creating barrier free environment specifying the modifications required regarding corridors, stairways, entrances, lightning or classroom arrangements so as to increase the level of accessibility. By observing the schools, it was revealed that more concrete and large-scale efforts must be made in this direction. Most of the schools did not possess many of the prescribed infrastructural standards. One of the major hurdles encountered by the visually challenged students had to do with gaining access to stairways and corridors. None of schools investigated had ramps for such special needs, which was supposed to be an essential requirement for schools integrating students with disabilities. Instead, all the schools had broad stairways with the maximum number of risers and inadequate handrails. This is in contrast to the guidelines specified in the Act. Moreover, the classrooms located on both sides of the corridor made it difficult for disabled children to access them comfortably, although some of the students were aware of their location and could access them with assistance from their fellow students. In addition to the classrooms, the location of the toilets, laboratories or cafeteria were also at a distance and required the students to travel across floors. All these factors restricted the mobility of the students with visual impairment, thus heightening their dependence on others. Furthermore, the classrooms did not have separate entrance and exit points. The seating arrangements also did not facilitate adequate mobility; specifically, tables and chairs were closely arranged, and there was no adequate space to facilitate easy movement. Moreover, most of the classrooms had inadequate lighting, and there was no arrangement through which students can store books, school bags and other personal items in school.

Regarding the educational aids and equipment in school for people with a disability, in all the three schools observed, most of the materials were not available. The students reported that the required materials, such as Braille writer, slate and stylus, magnification device and cassette tape recorder/player were not available in school. Moreover, the libraries did not have reading materials for the visually impaired students. This caused the students to depend on their sighted counterparts to read out to them; in certain cases, the students reported that they did not access the library at all. Though it is emphasised that use of models aimed at facilitating imparting of instruction, this facility was not found in any of the schools observed. The teaching was observed to be purely lecture-based theoretical in nature. Commenting on this issue, the concerned authorities, parents, and teachers held that the theoretical nature of the curriculum and work pressure prevent the students from continuing their studies on to the integrated schools. Under such circumstances, they often preferred the alternative schooling, i.e., National Institute of Open Schooling. This offers courses that have an advantage of being specially adapted to the needs of every child, thereby giving them the opportunity to progress at his/her own pace or join the community-based rehabilitation programmes. In view of these, it is maintained that despite the attempts towards integration, the efforts fail to meet the requirements of the ' basic ' curricular needs of these children, such as facilities for reading, writing, field trips, standards of attendance, participation, and so on.

The study was carried out by an NGO, All India Confederation of the Blind titled 'Assessment of Blindness Compensatory Skills among Visually Impaired Students of Class IV and V in Government Schools under SSA,' it was conducted among 200 visually impaired students across 10 states Bihar, Haryana, Madhya Pradesh, Rajasthan, Uttar Pradesh, Gujarat, Kerala, Maharashtra, Tamil Nadu and West Bengal.

The study revealed of all the 10 states, Gujarat ensured best care of its blind students, while it was found to be least as in case of Haryana, the least. Gujarat was found to indicate the highest state average in Braille writing, print writing and mathematics. Haryana and Bihar were reported to be the second worst wherein several zeros were reported in their scorecards. Apart from this the study also revealed scores of 200 students tested on their reading, writing and arithmetic skills using Braille or large print texts and tools like the abacus and Taylor frame. The students were divided into various categories of Blind, Very Limited Vision and Low Vision. The results were rather shocking since the average score was found to be 5.79 out of 25 (23.16 per cent) in Braille reading and 5.38 (21.52 per cent) in Braille writing. It was found to be more appalling for arithmetic on abacus, i.e., 2.59 (10.36 per cent) with the states of Bihar, Haryana, Kerala, Maharashtra and Rajasthan scoring zero and the rest not doing much better. The students were found to perform relatively well with an average of 64.4 per cent in Orientation and mobility.

5

Curriculum and Instructional Practices

Facing the Challenge of Curriculum Access and Instructional Practices

Physical facilities, technology, media and materials, and human resources all contribute to the quality of what transpires in schools. However, there yet remains great disparity in quality. To initiate any initiative the teachers inevitably need to ask a primary question to themselves: *what do my students need to know and be able to do?* To address these questions it is essential for the teachers to identify, locate, or develop curriculum—that which is generally believed to constitute the 'what' or substance of education for children with disabilities. This chapter will discuss possible adaptations to the curriculum, taking into account the children with visual impairment and with hearing impairment, their abilities and learning needs.

Curriculum and instructional practices cannot be easily separated conceptually from each other. However, in the present context, curriculum is treated as content and instruction is meant as those teaching practices that engage students in curriculum as disentangling the meaning of curriculum from instruction often proves unwieldy. Despite students with disabilities being classified into various categories, in most instances both the terms can be applied more generically. While students with complex healthcare issues, severe multiple disabilities and significant developmental may require approaches that offer intensive levels of support, students who are blind, deaf, deaf-blind, and autistic may in some cases require the same degree of support, but they also require more specialised curriculum and teaching approaches.

The curriculum essentially sets out what is to be taught, how it is to be taught and how learning is to be assessed. The fundamental issue for this review is how curriculum for students is designed, developed, delivered and assessed, with a focuss on the implications for students with special educational needs. At primary level, in many countries, students may be taught most or all subjects by the same teacher, in the same peer group and in the same classroom. Post-primary education often produces particular challenges for such students since the focuss at this stage is typically at subject rather than pupil/class level. This means that students with special educational needs may be taught in different peer groups for different subjects, by different teachers and in different geographical areas of a larger school. This tends to create challenges for students who find it hard to interact with their peers or who have issues with mobility or vision (Douglas et al, 2009).

Addressing the cause of education for the PWDs, the Persons with Disabilities Act specified that without prejudice to the foregoing provisions, the appropriate Governments shall by notification prepare a comprehensive education scheme which shall make provision for transport facilities to the children with disabilities or in the alternative financial incentives to parents or guardians to enable their children with disabilities to attend schools. Efforts would be made to the remove architectural barriers from schools, colleges or other institutions imparting vocational and professional training; supply books, uniforms and other materials to children with disabilities attending school; grant scholarship to students with disabilities; set up of appropriate for redressal of grievances of parents regarding the placement of their children with disabilities; make suitable modification in the examination system to eliminate purely mathematical questions for the benefit of blind students and students with low vision; restructure curriculum for the benefit of children with disabilities and restructure the curriculum for benefit of students with hearing impairment to facilitate them to take only one language as part of their curriculum. It also specified that all educational institutions shall provide amanuensis to blind students and students with or low vision.

Curriculum and Instructional Practices for Blind Students and Students with Low Vision

The curriculum for children with visual impairment is similar to the curriculum for sighted children and on the contrary it is more comprehensive. Apart from academic subjects, integration becomes effective when the student with visual impairment is well trained in compensatory skills such as Braille reading methods, use of slate and stylus, use of audio equipment, development of visual perceptual activities, speed and accuracy in the use of the abacus, skills of daily living and orientation and mobility. It is necessary for a resource teacher in consultation with the regular teacher needs to makenecessary changes in the presentation of materials in order to enable students to follow the general curriculum without any difficulty.

Students with blindness or low vision exhibit a wide range of visual impairments. It is important for the teachers to be aware that despite being diagnosed having the same eye condition and similar acuity no two students with low vision have the same functional vision. A myriad of factors such as fatigue, light glare, lighting conditions and time of day may influence vision and cause to fluctuate. Hence at the very outset, it is imperative to assess the needs of the student before necessary accommodations can be incorporated into his/her educational plan. This section highlights some of the guidelines for students with blindness and low vision at preschool, elementary and secondary levels. Students with visual impairments need the expanded core curriculum in addition to the core academic curriculum of general education. A quality education for students with disabilities will be a blending of curriculum designed to address disability-specific or unique needs and curriculum designed for optimal functioning in the mainstream society.

The Core Curriculum for Blind and Visually Impaired Children and Youths

Pre-school Blind or Visually Impaired

The preschool child who is blind or visually impaired may require direct teaching of skills and guidance through experiences which the child with normal vision encounters incidentally. The developmental progress of a child who is blind or visually impaired may be at the same rate as his or her sighted peers or may differ widely depending on a variety of factors such as degree of visual loss, age of diagnosis, presence or absence of additional disabilities, amount of early intervention or network of support available to the child and family. For Developmental Milestones for Infants with Visual Impairments refer to Appendix A.

In view of the fact that a child's vision may affect development, it is imperative that those working with the child should be aware of that visual diagnosis. The parents/guardians of a preschool child who is blind or visually impaired need to be informed of the child's specific individual visual impairment. Since children who are blind or visually impaired may lack a clear picture of their world this may necessitate assistance in all areas of their development: cognitive, linguistic, social, fine motor and gross motor. The focuss may be on helping them to acquire or learn new ideas/concepts through direct teaching. They may also need to supplement what they learn through vision by exploring their other senses as well. However, at the same time, it is important to keep in view that merely providing experiences to them is not enough. In doing so, one needs to keep in mind that the new experiences must be related to what the child's life and needs to be explained through a variety of techniques that would facilitate transfer of learning. There is the urgent need to provide detailed experiential teaching.

The curriculum for the preschool child must be developed based on the child's priority strengths and needs. Knowledge bases of team members (including parents) helps to provide various perspectives on the needs of the child. The curriculum should be child-specific with considerations for the visual impairment and the cognitive and physical needs of the child. The following are specific areas which must be considered when programming for the preschool child with a visual impairment:

- *Orientation and Mobility*: Efforts need to be made to familiarise the child with different environments.
- *Concept Development*: Since many concepts are to be taught to children who are blind or visually impaired through non-visual means and concrete experiences whenever possible it is advisable to use real objects. Experiences may need to be repeated many times and concepts should be taught in a variety of situations and in contexts that are meaningful to the child.
- *Sensory-Motor Skills*: Children who are blind or visually impaired will need direct teaching in sensory-motor skills in order to master interaction with their environment such as posture, head control, limb control, sitting, crawling, walking, balancing, grasping and holding objects, exploring objects tactually or differentiating between different textures.
- *Communication Skills*: There is the urgent need to identify the student's preferred modes of communication e.g., sign language, finger spelling, braille, speech or a combination of these. It is also important to identify that the student is able to receive and interpret was given through facial expressions, body language, gestures etc.
- *Daily Living Skills*: Training needs to be provided on self help skills for developing a sense of independence and self-esteem. Direct teaching will facilitate learning such skills such as eating, dressing, setting a table, brushing teeth and putting away toys.
- *Socialisation:* Children with visual impairment will require direct teaching of social skills so that they can learn acceptable ways of interacting with people and materials.

- *Technology and Special Equipment:* Children who are blind or visually impaired will learn early that technology is important to their lives and hence they should be exposed to computer technology as soon as possible and should begin to use tape recorders as a prelude to accessing books on audiotape. This learning can be combined with listening skills as well. Use of low vision aids such as magnifiers or telescopes can also be helpful.

Curriculum for the Elementary and Secondary Levels

The focuss being on inclusive education and child centered pedagogy necessitates that the curriculum to meet the needs of children with disabilities should also be suitably developed in consultation with experts so as to facilitate their inclusion with other children in regular classrooms. Regarding restructuring of curriculum for the benefit of children with disabilities particularly for dyslexic, blind, spastic and students with visual impairment, Section 30 of the Persons with Disabilities (Equal Opportunities, Protection of Rights and Full Participation) Act, 1995 stipulated certain modifications. It specified that dyslexic, blind, spastic and students with visual impairment have the option of studying one compulsory language as against two. The language opted by them should be in consonance with the overall spirit of the Three Language Formula prescribed by the Board. Besides one language, they can offer any four of the following subjects: Mathematics, Science and Technology, Social Science, Another Language, Music, Painting, Home Science and Introductory Information Technology.

Curriculum for blind children is never less than the curriculum for sighted children; on the contrary it is more comprehensive. In addition, for every skill expectation of the sighted child, blind children must do more. Apart from academic subjects, integration becomes effective when the blind child is well trained in compensatory skills such as Braille reading methods, use of slate and stylus, use of audio equipment, development of visual perceptual activities, speed and accuracy in the use of the abacus, skills of daily living and orientation and mobility. In order to enable the blind child to follow the general curriculum without any difficulty, the resource teacher, in consultation with the regular teacher, can make changes in the presentation of materials, if necessary. There are four principles involved in the preparation of materials:

- Duplication is the most encouraged method of materials preparation
- Modifications, in terms of content, method of display, type of material used, and the response expectation from the child, are sometimes made
- Sometimes, there is no suitable way to modify materials and therefore an experience may have to be substituted so that it closely approximates that presented to sighted counterparts.
- Under unavoidable circumstances, a concept or a lesson may have to be omitted.

The Existing Core Curriculum

- English language, arts, other languages, to the extent possible,
- Mathematics Science.
- Health, Physical Education.
- Fine Arts, Social Studies.
- Economics, Business Education.
- Vocational Education, History.

Hitchcock, Meyer, Rose, and Jackson (2002) define the general education curriculum as the overall plan for instruction adopted by a school or school system. They argued that blind students needed the same curriculum as every other student and that teachers could supply just a few additional skills and resources (Abel, 1959). These additional skills and knowledge areas became known as the 'plus curriculum.' Today, the plus curriculum is known as the 'expanded core' curriculum, to emphasise that it must go hand-in-hand with the 'common core' curriculum (Hatlen, 1996a). The expanded core curriculum is derived from the unique or disability-specific needs of blind and visually impaired students identified and elaborated by Hatlen and Curry (1987). The Table below is adapted from Hatlen (1996b).

The Expanded Core Curriculum

- Assistive technology/Technology.
- Career Education.
- Compensatory/Access Skills.
- Independent Living.
- Orientation and Mobility.
- Recreation and Leisure.
- Self-Determination.
- Sensory Efficiency.
- Social Interaction.

The following section provides a short description of the areas of expanded core curriculum. At the very outset in order to ensure greater understanding of the expanded core curriculum for blind and visually impaired students, it is imperative to consider the distinction between compensatory skills and functional skills. While mastery of compensatory skills enables by blind and visually impaired students to have access to learning in a manner equal to that of sighted peers as they are those needed in order to access all areas of core curriculum, Functional skills enable students with multiple disabilities to work, play, socialise, and take maximum care of their personal needs.

Compensatory and functional skills may include myriad of learning experiences such as concept development, spatial understanding, study and organisational skills, speech and listening skills, and adaptations essential for ensuring accessibility to all areas of the existing core curriculum. However, the instruction will be much dependent on the communication needs which vary depending on degree of functional vision, effects of additional disabilities and the task to be done. While this may necessitate some children to use braille, large print, print with the use of optical devices, while others may use regular print, tactile symbols, a calendar system, signlanguage, and/or recorded materials to communicate. Moreover, such an instruction also requires adequate expertise and professionalism in being prepared by the teachers. Unfortunately, they are not addressed with sufficient specificity in the existing core curriculum.

Unlike sighted children, acquisition of social interaction skills by blind and visually impaired individuals adults do not occur casually and incidentally. Rather, extreme care and organised efforts need to be taken while teaching them such skills so as to avoid social isolation.

Orientation and mobility also constitutes a vital area of learning and a part of the expanded core curriculum for blind and visually impaired learners. However, it is imperative that delivery of such a curriculum should be imparted by professionally trained and competent teachers. It is important for the students to acquaint themselves with their immediate and other associated environments. The existing core curriculum may fail to integrate these components in it and hence the expanded core curriculum must include emphasis on the fundamental need and basic right of visually impaired to develop optimum acquaintance with their environment.

Orientation and mobility skills contribute to development in social skills, mental and physical interactions and the general well-being of the student. These skills are needed for the student with low vision as well as the student with blindness. The amount of Orientation and Mobility training that a student will require depends on each student and how much vision he/she has. It should be incorporated into the student's programme plan and timetable. However, several factors need to be considered in determining an individual programme such as diagnosis and degree of visual impairment; prognosis of visual impairment; functional vision; presence of other disabilities; age; cognitive functioning; general health; school and community environment; and family, school and community resources.

Orientation skills can be incorporated within many regular classroom activities. Games, songs and activities can be used to teach or reinforce concepts such as body awareness and naming body parts, positional concepts, sensory awareness and basic movement patterns. Specific learning experiences planned for individual students can be taught and reinforced incidentally throughout the school day.

Creation of Environmental awareness may include awareness of air temperature, air currents, sun, scents, sounds, floor and wall coverings, furniture arrangement and objects in the hallway. Identification of landmarks may involve any permanent sensory information that assists an individual during independent travel. Location of rooms and flooring changes help students locate themselves within the school environment. Landmarks should have significance for the student. Identification of structural components of rooms and buildings can be imparted using models such as doll houses, Lego models and play house centres to help students understand concepts that they may not be able to experience visually. These may include corner, doorway, window, heating elements, basement, hallway, etc. Students also need to be acquainted with identification of directionality, i.e., left/right, followed by cardinal directions (north, south, east, west and interpretation of depth perception, i.e., coping skills to perceive relative distance of objects and their relationship to each other (stairs, curbs, terrain). To help the student understand his/her environment the teacher can point out environment symbols (signs, symbols, labels); point out objects in the environment so the student can make an association between the shape and its name; provide labels in the student's surroundings. Be sure, they are clear with good contrast; and teach the meaning of gestures and facial expressions to the student.

Mobility skills must be chosen in view of each student's specific needs and situation. Some of the common mobility skills which need to be taught include Sighted guide, Cane skills, Trailing, Self-protection, Search technique, Travel experience and Social skills. The students should be acquainted with the option of getting from place to place utilising the assistance of a sighted guide. For these teachers, staff, family members and peers can act as sighted guides and should be taught guide techniques. Regarding Cane skills once the need for the long white cane is determined, orientation and mobility instruction must commence to develop this highly essential and specialised skill. If the long white cane will be the eventual mobility device of choice, then it is imperative that a positive attitude for its use must be established early. Trailing can be demonstrated by extending one's arm at a 45 degree angle in front and to the side of the body, with the back of the hand following the trailing surface.

Self-protection techniques can be imparted by using either arm in combination with upper or lower protective techniques. In upper protective technique the arm is held across the upper body with the elbow bent and the palm facing forward. In the lower protective technique, the arm is held across the middle of the body with the elbow straight and the palm facing inward. In the Travel experience, a student should be made able to plan his/her route using tactile maps following simple routes using landmark sequencing and reverse directions to return to point of origin. The student should be able to travel within the home, school, neighbourhood, town and city. In order to accomplish this, the student will also need to be proficient at crossing a variety of streets. A student needs to develop travel routes such as home to school, quiet residential areas, small business areas, shopping areas, home to shopping areas and inside stores and businesses. The students also need to be acquainted with skills for using elevators and escalators, revolving doors, public transportation, travel in unknown areas and travel in adverse weather conditions.

Social skills need to equip students with, common courtesy in public, shopping skills, restaurant skills and phone resources for planning travel.

Besides orientation and mobility, another major area of concern for visually impaired learners is to develop in them self-independence in 'daily living skills.' Daily living skills essentially contain various tasks and functions which a person may need to perform such as personal hygiene, food preparation, money management, time monitoring, organisation, etc. in accordance with their abilities and independently. Keeping view of this, it can be mentioned that although some of these independent living skills are addressed in the existing core curriculum, but they often are introduced as piecemeal efforts. Such initiatives make it difficult to adequately prepare blind and visually impaired students for adult life.

Skills in recreation and leisure find little or no attention in the existing core curriculum. Although some emphasis is laid by way of physical education for the visually impaired learners in the form of team games there is absence of any conscious efforts for them to develop activities in recreation and leisure. Hence, well planned and deliberately taught expanded core curriculum should provide ample scope for teaching of recreation and leisure skills to blind and visually impaired students.

Since the desired outcome of life is preparation for independent living and to become a contributing member of the society, blind individuals are posed with several problems herein. There is a need for general vocational education, as offered in the traditional core curriculum, as well as the need for career education offered specifically for blind and visually impaired students. Many of the skills and knowledge offered to all students through vocational education can be of value to blind and visually impaired students. However, it is not sufficient to merely prepare students for adult life but instead career education as a part of the expanded core curriculum needs to provide the visually impaired learner across ages with the opportunity to acquire hands on experience as well as explore and develop their strengths and interests.

The opportunity to access and interact with text, both printed and electronic, continues to be fundamental in education for the visually impaired learners. It is essential that appropriate assistive technology enables students who are visually impaired to access information and to complete tasks efficiently enabling them to achieve the highest level of independence possible. Although in recent years assistive technology has enabled people with visual impairment to overcome stereotypes and to function efficiently in diverse professions of life much still needs to be done. Though training in assistive technology forms a part of the core curriculum, it being incorporated in the expanded core curriculum can ensure more concrete results. It is, however, important to bear in view that access to and instruction with assistive technology must be driven by individual needs, not by logistical constraints such as availability of equipment, location or model of service delivery, or funding restraints.

Significance of the Expanded Core Curriculum for Blind and Visually Impaired Students

Although it is undeniable that the existing core curriculum is essential to the learning of blind and visually impaired learners, it is equally irrefutable that the expanded core curriculum necessary for them. It is also a fact that though myriad of areas specified within the Expanded Core Curriculum for Blind and Visually Impaired Students is difficult to complete within the stipulated years prescribed for general education, this all the more necessitates the urgency for devising several approaches for incorporating the Expanded Core Curriculum into a normal course of education.

Moreover, since blind and low vision youngsters often do not bring the same visual experiences to the learning environment, it is very likely that their entire curriculum needs will not be met without planned, sequential, direct instruction by individuals who understand their learning style. In keeping view of this, it will be increasingly difficult expect that the competencies as reflected in the expanded core curriculum can be best achieved if infused within the existing, traditional curriculum. It is also important to bear in mind that it would indeed be difficult for visually impaired students to access both traditional and expanded core curriculum within the same time frame as their sighted counterparts there is lack of any single and simple method. At this time, no single, simple method has been developed that assures visually impaired students of accessing both traditional and expanded core curricula within the same time frame as their sighted peers.

In addition to these, it is imperative for the educators to overcome ignorance and become aware of the specialised needs of blind and visually impaired students. They need to develop professional skills and competencies for assessing, instructing, and evaluating unique and specialised curricular of visually impaired students. The educators for visually impaired students must adopt the expanded core curriculum based on the rationale that all students with visual impairments, including those with additional disabilities, have a fundamental right to an expanded core curriculum that emphasises students' opportunities to be equal and right to be different.

Fruitful implementation of the expanded core curriculum calls for equitable and focussed efforts and coordination among the educators, professionals and parent in preparing their children for a rich and fulfilling adult life.

Curriculum Suggestions for Teaching Students with Low Vision

This section highlights some of the aspects that need to be considered in providing instruction to students with low vision in different areas of the curriculum. Though the curriculum for students with low vision remains to be similar to their sighted counterparts, certain modifications need to be made to facilitate their better instruction. The section below discusses the curriculum for students with low vision with scope for certain modifications.

Teaching of Mathematics

It is important for students with low vision to learn how to physically manipulate concrete materials for mastering the basic concepts of mathematics. They need to acquire a thorough understanding of the basic concepts of addition, subtraction, multiplication and division before practicing on the abacus or talking calculator. They require greater practice of mental mathematics skills. A compartmentalised tray can be provided to them in which they can place articles for counting and matching. Pictorial directions can be useful for young students. It is necessary to demonstrate measuring instruments individually to the students and care needs to be taken to ensure that when doing activities involving measuring, the units used should be sufficientlylarge so that the student can work without assistance. The teacher needs to provide a worksheet instead of having the student copy from the board. The concept of money can be taught by making use of real coins while time through digital talking watches. Fractions can be taught to them through inlaid geometric puzzles can be useful for teaching fractions. Large print texts or the use of a closed circuit television can be especiallyhelpful in providing enlarged images of charts, diagrams, fractions and when teaching geometry.

Language teaching

As far as possible all objects in the room should be at the student's eye level and the teacher needs to point out details in pictures to aid with comprehension. Templates or line guides can help a student focuss on what they're reading. Adjustable reading stands can promote good reading posture and reduce neck and back fatigue. More emphasis should be placed on vocabulary building, word-attack skills andcomprehension rather than speed. Large print is not necessary for all students with low vision and often normal print held close to the eyes is legible. Oral drills in particular help to improve the student's spelling. Paper with well-spaced bold black lines is useful for printing and handwriting. The students should also be introduced to keyboarding skills by grade three or four.

Teaching of Social Studies

Raised line, large print or bold line maps and atlases can be useful for the students. Reference materials may be scanned and listened to on a computer with voice access to decrease the amount of reading required.

Teaching of Science

Raised line, large print or bold line diagrams can be useful for the students and it is necessary to avoid too much of detail. The students may also need assistance in a laboratory to describe changes and aid in measurement. The student should be allowed to examine the apparatus and materials before and then experiment. If possible some of the science equipments can be available with tactile markings. It can be beneficial if real life articles or models are used.

Unique Curriculum Needs for Students with Low Vision

Although a student with low vision can participate in the regular school programme with adaptations it is also important to provide them with more directed instruction in the following areas than a child with normal vision:

- Visual efficiency;
- Concept development;
- Listening skills;
- Knowledge of the eye condition;
- Sensory-motor skills/physical education;
- Visual aids and adaptations;
- Communication;
- Orientation and mobility;
- Self-concept and socialisation;
- Daily living skills;
- Career education;
- Recreation and leisure; and
- Sex education.

Both the resource and classroom teachers need to coordinate in the development and implementation of the student's programme. To facilitate this they need to hold regular meetings with the support team, particularly those who will be working directly with the student and discuss daily, weekly or long-range programme plans.

Curriculum Suggestions for Teaching Students with Visual Impairment and Other Disabilities

Visual impairments may exist among students along with developmental disabilities, deafness or hard of hearing, or physical disabilities. In such instances it is imperative to assess each disability separately and to assess how the combined disabilities impact the student's total performance. Coping effectively with such students necessitates a coordinated interdisciplinary team approach to assessment and programme planning among occupational and physiotherapists; speech and language pathologists; social workers; and others.

Instructional Practices for Students with Visual Impairments and Developmental Disabilities

The instructional process must include opportunities for the student to explore new objects and places and be exposed to a variety of experiences. Students must experience a variety of textures, shapes, weights, temperatures, sounds, smells and tastes to build meaningful relationships and concepts about the environment. Opportunities need to be provided to practice and reinforce skills in natural settings throughout the day. Repetition enables the student to master new skills. Use of tactile, concrete and real life material provides opportunities for kinesthetic and tactile learning. If a student has residual hearing, use of stationary sound sources helps to orient the student regarding important locations and landmarks. The instructor needs to ensure that activities should be task analysed and broken down into steps so that each step can be taught sequentially. The instructional process should also enable the student to develop meaningful relationships with adults and peers who may or may not have disabilities.

6

Assistive Technology

Role of Assistive Technology for Blind Students and Students with Low Vision

In the age of incessant technological advancement, there is tremendous demand for incorporation of new and modern programmes and methods in order to ensure greater adaptability with the pace of rapid competition. The same holds true for people with disabilities all over the world. Visualisation which is regarded an inevitable medium for people to adapt to complex information as well as to navigate around structured information; the visually challenged are placed at a vulnerable position by nature. However, the situation seems to be undergoing rapid and more positive changes with the ushering in of new technological interventions.

The opportunity to access and interact with text, both printed and electronic, continues to be fundamental to education in the information age. Appropriate assistive technology has enabled students who are visually impaired to access information and to complete tasks efficiently enabling them to achieve the highest level of independence possible. Emerging research suggests that technology promotes acquisition of literacy, provides more equal access to information required for employment, and for access to information, in general, and facilitates social and community networks (Kelly and Smith, 2011). In recent years, assistive technology has enabled people with visual impairment to overcome stereotypes and to function efficiently in diverse professions of life.

The most important advancement since blind assistive technology began to appear in the 1970s is the screen reading software, which simulates the human voice reading the text on computer screen or renders hard-copy output into Braille. Screen reading software such as JAWS, Job access with Speech, by Freedom Scientific, Window-Eyes by GW Micro, and Serotek are being used widely by the visually impaired students to read the text appearing on the screen. Their ease in operation by keyboard commands and the options of Braille display and a synthetic voice facilitates better instruction. Given the current state of technologies for displaying refreshable braille or magnified text, paired with speech driven by screen reader technology, students can now access information available in text through multiple modalities. The optical character recognition which scans and reads the text aloud has enabled students with visual impairments to access all types of print materials by using this scanning technology. Portable reading devices are now being used to download books and read them out loud in a synthesised voice such as the Victor Reader Stream and the Book Sense.

The apparent benefits of Audio Supported Reading (ASR) suggest that rather than teaching the skills essential for braille reading, print reading, and listening in isolation as separate pedagogies, a more robust and integrated approach for teaching and acquiring literacy skills will be more advantageous. In today's era of general curriculum access and high stakes testing, it is imperative that new practices and pedagogies be examined with a view to improving results for these students, many of whom lag far behind their typically sighted counterparts. In addition to computers and other devices, talking clocks and thermometres, specialised bar code scanners, and palm pilots all make daily life, education and employment more accessible for people with vision impairment. The GPS system including Braille

Note GPS, Street Talk™, Trekker, and Mobile GEO have also taken a lead in facilitating mobility of people with visual impairment.

A broad range of devices from 'low tech' such as markers, paper stabilisers to 'high tech' such as Braille readers, computers, etc., are included among the assistive technology devices. However, the uses of technology by students who are blind or visually impaired largely depend on their own personal desires as well as availability of requirements. The section below discusses some of the technological aids that can be used by the visually challenged individuals. Technological equipment for the visually challenged or the blind primarily falls into two categories: non-electronic and electronic.

The Non-electronic equipment includes a wide variety of objects such as the Dark-Line paper, Non-carbonised (NCR) Paper, Braille Paper and Paper Holders, Large Print or Braille Textbooks and Novels, Mathematical Aids, Reading Stands, Abacus, Tactile Maps and Diagrams, Science Aids, Raised Line Drawing Kit, Braille Compass, Slate and Stylus, Braille Writer, Low Vision Aids, etc.

The Electronic equipment includes Calculator, Electronically Enlarged Material, Four-Track Tape Recorder, Textbooks and Novels on Tape, Electronic Dictionary with Speech, Closed Circuit Television (CCTV), Portable Note Takers, Laptop Computers, Speech Synthesisers and Screen Reading Software, Text Enlarging Software, Optical Character Recognition (OCR) System, Braille Translation Software, Braille Embosser, etc.

Non-electronic Equipment

- *Braille Writer*: The Perkins Braille Writer is a non-electronic device used to produce braille material and can be used for both long and short braille work.

- *Slate and Stylus*: The slate is a small metal or plastic device in two pieces, hinged together. The bottom piece is flat, while the top piece has several rows of braille cells. The student places paper between the two pieces and uses the stylus, a small pointed instrument, to produce braille by pressing the correct dots in the braille cells. A braille letter or letter group is embossed on the paper which can then be read by the student.

• *Computational Aids*: The Taylor slate was one of the earliest manipulative/tactile aids used with the visually impaired students of mathematics. It measures about 11 by 17 inches, has a tray to hold pegs and an array of holes about 22 of them across and about 20 holes in a column to contain these pegs. These holes are shaped similar to a plus sign overlying an 'X' and the pegs have the same shape. At each end of the one inch pegs, to one side, is a bar and at the other end two conical projections. The angle of insertion determines the numerical value, with the bar side up the positions run one through 8 and flipping the pegs over the values 9 and 0, with the remainder of the positions determining the operation.

Later, the Brannan slate was used which consists of a 16 by 16 array of square holes that hold small dice-like cubes which have raised Braille numbers. The position of the cube determines which Braille number is being used while one side of the cube indicates the operation thus enabling the blind children to set up their own problems.

• *Graphing Aids*: Graphing aids for the blind or visually-impaired student are of a wide variety ranging from embossed Braille paper to graphing utilities that can access a tactile printer which provides raised-line drawings.

• *The Embossed Braille Paper:* Contains grids ranging from 1/2 to 1-inch which are mounted by the student onto cork boards. Push pins help to locate the coordinates and are connected with rubber bands (Garvin 1994). A teaching aid called Wacky Sticks, made of wax in long strips, can be also be used with the embossed Braille paper. These strips can be broken into small dots to represent points on a graph.

• *Sewell Raised-line Drawing Kit*: This kit consists of a clipboard with a rubber pad, stylus, and Mylar sheets. A Mylar sheet is inserted under two thumbscrews, and then the stylus is used to create a picture. A raised line is formed because of the stretching capability of the thin Mylar.

• *Other Mathematical Aids*: Dark and/or raised-line rulers, raised clock faces, geometric volume and area aids, braille protractors, Braille compasses, braille rulers and braille tape measures.

• *Low Vision Aids*: Low vision aids include magnifying glasses and telescopic aids. The magnifiers may be hand—held, sitting on the material or attached to eyeglasses helping the student complete near distance tasks such as reading or writing. The Telescopic aids are used for seeing material at a distance and may be either hand-held or attached to eyeglasses.

Advent and Evolution of Braille in India

Genesis of Braille System in India could be traced back to Miss Hewlett who, at a very young age, lost her vision for a year and regained it after a successful eye operation. It was Miss Hewlett, a Christian Missionary, in1879 or a little later, who invited and requested one more young Christian Missionary, Miss Annie Sharp to receive requisite training in special education to teach the blind of this country who were living in a piteous and sorrowful situation. Catching an inspiration from Miss Hewlett, Annie Sharp on her return to India from Perkins set up a North India Industrial Home for the Christian Blind at the Saint Catharine Hospital in Amritsar on 1887. It was the first school for the blind in India. Thus, Miss Annie Sharp became the 'Mother of educational facilities for the blind, in India'. Doctor Neelkanth Rai Dahiyabhai Chatrapati, even before launching his own co-ed school for the Blind at Ahmedabad in 1895, went to Annie Sharp's school at Amritsar and received training in Braille. Doctor Neelkanth Rai Dahiyabhai Chatrapati lost his vision adventitiously and even then, he worked tirelessly to evolve a common Braille code for India. L. Garth Waite in unison with Reverend J. Knowles developed Oriental Braille and brought it to India at around the same time when Annie Sharp opened her first school in 1887. But Lal Bihari Shah learnt Braille from L. Garth Waite in 1893 and developed his own Braille code, effecting certain changes in the original Braille System invented by the genius of Louis Braille. His code later went on to be evolved into the Bangla Braille Code. Lal Bihari

Shah also strongly advocated the need for a common Braille code for the whole country. Subsequently, P.M. Advani also evolved Sindhi Braille Code, but kept always striving for a burning necessity for a common code for the country.

Apart from these luminaries of Braille World in India, many other veterans thought and worked hard to evolve a common Braille code for Indian languages. Thus, by the year 1947 when India gained its freedom, there were ten different Braille codes being used in different schools for the blind across the country which were as follows:

- Tamil Braille of Miss Askwith;
- Oriental Braille by Reverend J. Knowles and Mr L. Garth Waite;
- Shah Braille Code;
- Indian Braille of Doctor Neelkanth Rai Dahiyabhai Chatrapati;
- Mysore and Kannada Code;
- Sindhi Braille Code of Mr P.M. Advani;
- Shirreff Braille;
- Chatterjee Braille Code;
- Uniform Indian Braille Code framed by the Expert Braille Committee of the Central Advisory Board of Education; and
- Standard Indian Braille Code framed by an Informal Committee under the Chairmanship of Lt. Col. Sir Clutha Mackenzie, the commandant, Saint Dunstun's Hostel for Indian War Blinded, which later culminated in to NIVH.

From this all, one can conclude that before 1951, when Bharati Braille was finally drawn up, the education of visually impaired children was pervaded by chaos and confusion and the net result was the total disaster in education of the visually impaired.

Electronic Equipment

- *Braille Translation Software:* Converts text to Braille ready to be printed on a Braille Embosser. Translated text may then be printed for the student using a braille embosser (braille printer). Braille translation software may be included as a programmeon a student laptop computer

- *Braille Embosser*: The braille embosser is a printer attached to a computer which is used to produce a braille copy of text. It may also be attached to braille note taking devices for the same purpose. This can enable a student to print a copy of his or her personal notes and written work.

- *Speech Synthesisers and Screen Reading Software*: This hardware and software enable students who are blind are to aurally access print material on a computer screen. They can use the Internet, word processing programs, calculators and access other printed material without having to see the screen.

- *Computational Softwares*: Software packages, used in conjunction with an adapted computer, have enhanced accessibility for the visually impaired. Most have scientific functions including trigonometric, logarithms, exponents, and roots. All entries, functions and answers are spoken. These are available through the Internet at various FTP sites.

Another software package converts the computer-like system of Braille-n-Speak 640S and Type-n-Speak. This shareware alters these notepads into scientific calculators.

- *The Nomad Pad* is an interactive audio-tactile graphics system developed in Australia. This touch pad enables a student to study a series of prepared graphs independently. However, it does not allow blind/visually-impaired students to create their own graphics.

- *Screen Readers (Text to Speech)*: It is an alternative to standard computer output where the computer 'reads' text on the standard display to the user. The Speech output can range from computers with sound cards that can read text to a fully functional screen reading package such as talking web browsers.

- *Portable Note Takers*: Portable note taking devices may be used by a student to take notes in class using either a braille or standard keyboard which may then be transferred to a computer for storage, or printed in either braille or print formats. This is very effective for certain applications, for example word-processing. Many note taking devices have word processors, appointment calendars, calculators or clocks, etc.

• *Braille Keyboards*: A braille input keyboard can be connected to either the serial or keyboard ports on a PC. It can mimic every key on a full standard keyboard but may only allow the input of Grade one Braille. However, its main application is often limited to programmers using terminal emulation software.

• *Haptic Devices*: These two-dimensional devices are used to provide a slight resistance at the edges of windows and buttons so that the user can 'feel' the Graphical User Interface (GUI) and 'feel' pictures such as maps and drawings by providing resistance to textures in computer images.

• *Scanners with Optical Character Recognition*: Character recognition software can convert scanned documents into machine-readable print, large print, Braille and synthetic speech.

• *Four-Track Tape Recorder*: The recorder allows the student to hear material which is recorded on two tracks per each side of a regular cassette tape.

• *Closed Circuit Television (CCTV)*: Magnification systems based on closed circuit cameras are used to produce an enlarged image of text on a monitor or TV. A camera is used to project the image of the printed material onto a television screen at the student's eye level. With this equipment, the student is able to view print material of all types as well as charts, diagrams and photographs.

Now since much has been mentioned about the use of computers in the education programme of the visually challenged the question arises as to how does a blind person use a computer:

There are two basic approaches:

- Everything that appears on the screen, also appears on the 'screen for the blind', so called Braille display. It is a row of Braille letters which the blind can read (feel).
- Everything that happens on the screen is being read or vocally reproduced so the computer programmetells them what is on the screen. Programmes that are used for

adaptation of the screen content for vocal or Braille reproduction are called screen readers.

Sometimes, these two approaches are also usually combined so that the users of Braille display sometimes listen to the screen content and on other times can read using the display. Currently keeping view of the voluminous size, sensitivity and complexity of the mainframe computer, recent advances in technology of the transistor and silicon chip have promoted the use of micro-computers.

Orientation and Mobility Aids

Besides the use of technological aids for educational purposes of the students, it is also of equal importance to offer assistance in orientation and mobility. The broad domain of orientation and mobility can include certain structural adaptations, fabrications in the home, worksite or other area (ramps, lifts, bathroom changes) that remove or reduce physical barriers for an individual with a disability. With the objective of structural adaptations in view in the Indian context, The Persons With Disabilities (Equal Opportunities, Protection of Rights and Full Participation Act), 1995 emphasised upon removal of architectural barriers from schools, colleges or other institutions imparting vocational and professional training. It detailed out the architectural and instructional barriers and specified the need for each institute to identify the type of infrastructure to be / modified for enabling the government to provide financial assistance for such upgradation/modification and laid down detailed guidelines for creating barrier-free environment specifying the modifications required regarding corridors, stairways, entrances, lightning, classroom arrangements etc. thereby increasing the level of accessibility.

Traditionally, a blind person relied on a guide dog or a long cane to navigate the environment. However, the last thirty years have witnessed engineers devoting considerable resources for developing electronic systems to help a blind person avoid obstacles. Several electronic mobility aids have been developed such as the use of ultrasonics; as with radar in which the range is obtained from the length of time, it takes for a pulse to be reflected back to the transceiver while other systems use lasers or infra-red.

- *Sonic Pathfinder*: This is a head-mounted device which provides a simple tonal display that provides advance warning of objects that lie in the user's travel path. It is a highly selective aid, providing information only of immediate practical use to the pedestrian and prioritising objects lying straight ahead of the user.
- *Long Cane*: It is usually made of hollow, light-weight, aluminum alloy. The nylon cane tip is designed to transmit tactual information up through the cane.

Embossed maps can also be used to help a visually person to get acquainted with the layout of the environment.

Issues and Challenges

Although the need for and benefit of assistive technology has been well-documented throughout literature, there are various complex issues that often restricts the use of assistive technology devices and software. One such problem centres on the fact that most of the provision of assistive technology are not based on the particular needs of individual but upon disability. There is frequent ignorance of the fact that even students with the same visual loss may require instruction in different types of assistive technology based upon their unique needs. Besides this, it is also imperative to take into account that determination of access mode(s), i.e., speech access, braille access, print access, tactile communication systems etc. and must be guided by skilled specialists in the education of students with visual impairments who have comprehensive expertise in blindness and low vision specific assistive technology and who can also access individual learning characteristics.

There is also the need to diagnose the specific needs of students with visual impairments followed by proper planning, implementation, and continuous monitoring instruction in the use of appropriate technology. Students with visual impairments will not be included unless their unique educational needs for access are addressed by specially trained personnel in appropriate environments and unless these students are provided with equal access to core and specialised curricula through appropriate specialised books, materials and equipments. Hence, it is imperative that efforts must be directed towards appropriate instruction including designing a plan of individualised assistive technology instruction and teaching a specialised hierarchy of skills that is based upon diagnostic evaluations. Instruction in the use of appropriate assistive technology devices such as speech, large print, Braille must take place concurrently with instruction in keyboarding, word processing, and use of the Internet. Appropriate instruction also needs to be provided concerning introduction to or mastery of other blindness and low vision specific assistive technology devices such as electronic note takers, scanners, optical character recognition (OCR) systems, braille translation software, braille and print embossers, screen magnification software, etc.

Access to and instruction with assistive technology must be driven by individual needs, not by logistical constraints such as availability of equipment, location or model of service delivery, or funding restraints. Currently, some students with visual impairments have access to a wide range of blindness and low vision specific assistive technology devices, while others have none at all (Kelly, 2008). In inclusive classrooms, students with disabilities do not always have access to the same learning tools as their classmates. For instance, while the students with visual impairments have to rely on alternative-format books, such as large print or Braille as compared to their sighted counterparts who access written text, the former are dependent on their teachers and peers to describe the matter to them and also in certain cases visual materials may never be adapted. Moreover, though use of educational software has become an important tool and their use is continuously being emphasised on in classrooms it poses certain challenges for the students with disabilities. For instance, while a sighted student can learn a biology lesson based on interactive simulation, a student with low vision may have to depend on assistive interactive software for experimental. Though the accessible software can contribute positively toward filling in some of the gaps resulting from lack of exposure to a wide range of activities the issue of proper accessibility and training becomes important.

According to the 2009 WHO fact sheet, there are 314 million visually-impaired people worldwide and 87 per cent of them live in developing countries. Forty five million people are classified as blind of whom, the majority belongs to India. In India, blind children may attend regular public schools where both visually impaired and non-visually impaired students are integrated or residential schools created specifically for the visually impaired. Although several technology aids are available to visually impaired people in developed countries, due to high cost, these tools are often not accessible to people in developing communities. Furthermore, most schools in developing communities who have advanced technology such as a braille embosser receive the technology through donations.

One specific instance of this difference is that wealthier schools possessing many teaching aids for visual concepts enable blind students to build a strong sense of shapes and tactile perception of images thus experiencing the world using sensors other than vision. These educational tools range from plastic molds, to embossed maps, and image-embossing printers. They are used to teach subjects such as mathematics, geography, physics and biology, in which sighted people take images, maps, and diagrams for granted. Diagrams, charts, graphs, maps, and other non-verbal displays are encountered increasingly in all educational materials. The ability to understand these graphics is becoming expected of all educated adults.

There is significant desire for images in the school's curriculum. The teachers explained their difficulties in teaching subjects like mathematics, science, and geography especially when trying to explain shapes, diagrams, maps, and the human anatomy. When local-language textbooks are translated into braille, pictures are omitted and references to them are deleted. In the first and second grades, images of basic shapes are removed and figures are omitted. In the seventh grade, pictures of internal organs such as the brain, lungs, and heart are omitted. In the tenth grade, students learn history and geography without the aid of maps. Due to this, the students only learn to recite the words of their teachers. Lack of access to images results in students memorising facts as verbal assertions, without associating them to concrete mental images. Arguing that since students find it extremely difficult to understand the image and graph-rich curricula in advanced mathematics and science, most schools in India do not include mathematics and science after the seventh grade and emphasise exclusively on teaching humanities.

Instruction by qualified educational professionals is often hindered by lack of pre-service and in-service training in assistive technologies. It is evident from research that some students with visual impairments have access to teachers who are well-prepared to deliver special instruction in blindness and low vision specific assistive technology, while others do not (Abner and Lahm, 2002; Edwards and Lewis, 1998; Kapperman, Sticken and Heinze, 2002; Murphy, Hatton and Erickson, 2008; Parker et al., 1990; Sahfi, Zhou, Smith and Kelley, 2009; Smith, Kelley, Maushak, Griffin-Shirley and Lan, 2009). Hence, there is the urge to eliminate this inequity. Opportunities must be provided for professional development through partnerships among school, universities, organisations as well as assistive technology vendors to ensure that professionals keep abreast of emerging technologies.

Factors such as location, cost, and personnel often hinder the availability of assistive technologies for individuals with visual impairments. The main problems are not only associated with designing the electronic circuitry for a satisfactory electronic mobility aid but in identifying the optimum information needed for independent traveling, displaying this information to the blind persons in a non-visual format, i.e., auditory or vibratory signals, manufacturing the device at a reasonable price and finally training of the blind persons in the use of these devices. Referring to issue of structural adaptations for effective orientation and mobility of the visually challenged as well as other forms of disabilities most of the schools in India do not possess many of the prescribed infrastructural standards as specified by the 1995 Persons With Disability Act. There is still lack of basic requirements such as ramps, adequate Braille books, etc. Moreover, though embossed maps can be used in familiarising a visually challenged person with the layout of the environment they are not easy to produce or interpret since just embossing a sighted map may not ensure an intelligible embossed map.

Limited awareness among non-specialist sighted users about the difficulties encountered by the visually impaired users in adapting to the new technology such as investing a great deal of time in learning the command structure and operation of the speech, Braille, or text display system can further hinder in providing assistance. Hence, attempt should be made towards providing structured training so as to bring positive benefits to those who need to use technology for a specific range of tasks.

Implications for Practice

Effort needs to be directed towards making the various products more accessible. This is important because in certain occasions the educational goals of a programme are sometimes incompatible with providing non-visual access for students who are blind. Moreover, many programme may emphasise on teaching visual concepts, such as counting and colour-pattern matching using only visual ways of teaching which blind students may find difficult to access. Though students with low-vision may learn from a visual programme, it is essential for it to be well designed such as the software should allow fonts to be adjusted, provide clear contrast for objects that students can locate and manipulate, include keyboard commands to reduce mouse dependence and provide a system cursor that moves with important screen events so that magnifiers can track them.

There is the need to consider the age and skills of the students in developing the educational software for the students. For instance, a young child with visual impairment may be comfortable with software that may require a teacher to set options for them, such as enhanced audio, larger fonts and icons, and high contrast backgrounds while the older students may need to use a screen magnifier and therefore, rely less on adjustments available within the programme itself. Besides this, it is important to consider the amount of experience and comfort a person has in using software. While some visually challenged students may feel more competent and confident having received keyboard training in advance, others may prefer using their assistive technology only for rudimentary tasks. In view of the above said, the range of skills, comfort levels and technology limitations should be considered in deciding accessibility to educational softwares.

Accessible textbooks and software often provide multi-modal access to information, combining text with audio. Hence providing accessible electronic publications, such as textbooks, journals or training materials, can help to bridge the gap for students who depend on the use of adapted materials.

It is believed that good design practice, mobility training and relevant assistive devices can help people to become independently mobile. Hence, efforts need to be made in this direction to ensure a blend of all the above three. With this objective in view certain initiatives need to be undertaken such as any design or technological changes made to an environment must be carried out in such a manner so that it benefits the full range of independently mobile blind and partially sighted people. Comprehensive mobility training needs to be provided which can enable the user to move safely. However, in doing so, good building design and good environment design can make this process easier. Regarding use of good design practice which can make buildings easier to be used by blind and partially sighted people, certain information required could be directional information such as for the library turn left and for the school office turn right, etc. Attempts can be made to provide such information via a push button sign or a tactile sign. However, since both the signs would require the blind or partially sighted user to know that a sign is available and their approximate position a remotely triggered audible sign can be designed to provide the information to the user easily.

Conclusion

Lowenfeld (1973) determined that there were three primary issues facing individuals with visual impairments: access to information, independent travel and lack of meaningful experiences. Assistive technology is used by individuals with visual impairments to compensate for these limitations, achieve educational success, gain competitive employment by providing tools for increased independent access to information and for effective communication. The current challenge is to provide appropriate access to and instruction on blindness and low vision specific assistive technology through individualised assessment of assistive technology needs, appropriate instruction in the use of assistive technology as tools and equitable distribution of assistive technology.

With progress and preparation for a prosperous future being the chief goal in today's world, Cage (1984) had rightly stated, 'We [educators] are a profession that serves, but yet leads students into a challenging and ever changing tomorrow'. With this objective in view, it is essential for the educational leaders to emerge out of the existing boundaries and explore new horizons. They need to develop/design, redesign as well as implement new and more developed assistive devices and programmes for the visually challenged. This eventually would not only prepare the visually challenged individuals for the technocratic world but also ensure their integration into the mainstream society.

7

Teachers: Aproach, Attitudes and Roles

Teachers Role and Approach

The fundamental importance of teachers' position in the process of learning is simply undeniable. Their expectations, sensitiveness, priorities and values contribute to the quality of pupils' learning experiences and consequently they influence what id taught, how it is taught and the assessment of what has been taught (Harnett and Naish, 1993). Similarly, the attitude of teachers has been regarded as one of the factors guaranteeing the success of integration of students with special needs.

Teachers' attitude towards students with disabilities depends on several factors: nature of the society, prevailing conceptions of disability, teachers' age, grade, training, teaching experience with individuals. Moreover, Combs and Harper (1967) found that the use of labels, per se, affects the attitudes of teachers towards children with disabilities, but is inconsistently dependent on the type of disability.

Researchers have portrayed a mixed attitude on the part of teachers towards children with disabilities per se and the blind in specific. Researchers like Hayes and Gunn (1988) and Thomas

(1985) indicated that teachers hold negative attitude towards children with disabilities. They found to associate the presence of such children in their class with trouble (Pastor and Jimenez, 1994). They hold that placing such children in the class would result in disparity of level between pupils and that it would hinder the pace of the course. Moreover, catering to children with disabilities requires extra time and effort which would take teaching away from other children since instruction in the regular classroom is based on standard progress of sighted children (Miller and Switzerkey, 1978; Diamond, 1979; Bulliole and Rigg, 1980). The teachers were further found to hold that lack of flexibility and responsiveness to the needs of children with disabilities and the restrictive approach to education makes it difficult to organise learning experiences that promote social interaction among such children and their sighted counterparts. Another factor has been observed that while teachers have been actively involved in the integration process, they recognised the necessity of providing for different levels of learning within classrooms with special emphasis still continuing to be placed on resourcing of special needs rather than on changing pedagogical practices. Such difficulties tend to create a sense that within one classroom there are two types of teachers and two different groups of children (Johnson and Johnson, 1980; Schopler and Bristol, 1980).

In view of such a situation, teachers tend to prioritise their responsibilities, leaning more towards the normal children and view integrated educational practices as an additional burden. Hence, they do not regard integration of such children to be a concern of theirs but perceive it to be a political and administrative problem, which should be met by physical measures. Alves and Gottlieb (1986) observed teacher interaction with students with and without disabilities. On analysis, it was revealed that students with disabilities received few questions and were provided with less teacher feedback than their normal classmates indicating that children with disabilities were less involved in academic exchanges.

Research has also indicated an emerging trend of positive attitude on the part of regular teachers (Whinnery, Fuchs and

Fuchs, 1991; Wood, 1992). Some of the regular educators have displayed enthusiastic professional dedication to the development and implementation of inclusive school practices. It was found that greater contact with children with disabilities enabled teachers to gain greater insight into their needs and problems. Clarity of views coupled with necessary assistance and training also helped them to develop favourable attitudes.

Rogers (1951) developed a teacher and student-centred approach. He maintained that students have a capacity for self-awareness, self-understanding and self-direction, for growth and constructive change. This approach was found to be suitable for the visually impaired children. According to him, students structure themselves according to their perception of reality. Rogers (1967) mentioned six characteristics necessary and sufficient for change or growth to take place in students: Two people are in psychological contact with each other; one (student) is in a state of incongruence, vulnerable or anxious, ready for change; the other (teacher) is congruent; the teacher possesses and exhibits unconditional positive regard for the student; the teacher possesses and exhibits empathetic understanding of the students' internal frame of reference and the student becomes aware of and experiences unconditional positive regard and empathetic understanding.

Rogers also mentioned that it was essential for the teacher to possess certain characteristics in order to bring about a positive impact on the self-esteem of blind students: reflects the content and feelings expressed by student; clarifies students' messages; assists students' understanding through teacher's self-disclosure, engages in 'you-me' talk that is concrete and specific, especially about personal attributes, aspirations, beliefs and standards and values; confronts whenever necessary as an invitation for the students to examine discrepancies; helps students master his own resource and encourages students to find his own solutions. Hence, the teacher should display qualities of empathy, understanding as well as allow students to undergo experiences, learn to trust in themselves, develop an internal locus of control and willingness to make choices or decisions.

Savage and Weinke (1990) conducted a study to determine teachers' attitude towards mainstreaming. Two hundred and eighty one responses were obtained from 119 primary, 98 intermediate and 64 secondary teachers who responded to a teacher opinion survey. The relationship between frequency contact (FC), teacher experience (TE) and teacher level (TL) was determined. Teacher experience was found to correlate significantly with teacher level and a small but significant positive relationship was found between attitude and frequency of contact with the resource teacher. Findings also revealed a trend for secondary teachers to be less accepting than other teachers of special needs students in regular class. Witter (1990) in a study involving one hundred and nineteen children and twenty teachers from residential schools for children with emotional and bahavioural difficulties found that strategies associated with lack of structure and control, with permissiveness and instant material rewards were perceived by all students to be associated with low self-esteem and least likely to improve it.

Murphy (1960) asked several educators to rank categories of exceptional children according to those they would most prefer to teach and those they most understood. It was found that majority of the respondents only placed the blind children on the rejection end of the continuum but also signified that they knew very little about these children in comparison to those having other types of disability. Schmidt and Nelson (1968) while studying the attitude of special teachers towards cognitive and affective goals for the blind students found that their goals were more cognitive than the regular teachers but their attitudes were negative. Kuhn (1971) pointed out that teachers in an elementary school had a resource room for blind students and those who had constant contact with those students did not hold significantly different attitudes, i.e., had negative attitude towards the students as compared to the teachers from another elementary school who did not have any contact with them.

Pliner and Hannah (1985) while studying teachers attitude towards four types of children with disabilities (visual, hearing, orthopaedically and emotionally disturbed) found negative attitude only when a child's level of achievement was low and not due to their placement. Alves and Gottlieb (19860 observed teacher interaction with students with and without disabilities and on analysis found that students with disabilities received few questions, were provided with less teacher feedback than their counterparts and were less involved in academic exchanges.

Pastor and Jimenez (1991) while investigating the position of blind students in regular schools and teachers' perspective on their integration found negative attitude.

Buthrow et al (1998) investigated the ratings of regular teachers and parents of the social skills of blind students aged six to ten years from grades one to five along with sighted children. The study revealed that the teachers rated the blind students lower in cooperation, academic competence and as having greater problem behaviour than the sighted counterparts. Glaubman and Lifshitz (2001) undertook study to investigate the attitude of teachers in the independent educational system of the Haredi community towards the inclusion of pupils with special needs in the regular classrooms. The results revealed unwillingness of teachers to include blind and deaf pupils in their classes.

As against Kuhn's argument Keilbaugh (1975) undertook a study with thirty-one elementary school teachers to determine their attitude towards blind students in integrated settings and a questionnaire containing seventeen items were administered. The results indicated positive attitude on the part of the teachers with little difference between teachers who had previous exposure to special education course work and those who had none.

The classroom teacher of a student who is blind or visually impairedneeds to undertake certain initiatives to facilitate better instruction and social rehabilitation. However, it is important to bear in mind that although all suggestions provided may not directly relate to all students, an overview certainly will ensure positive desired results:

- If any teacher suspects that a child has a problem with vision needs to refer him/her for screening to a school medical officer. It is important to identify the students for providing proper help (See Appendix B and Appendix C). A medical certificate and a File Review Form can be maintained concerning each child (See Appendix D and E for a sample).

- The teachers can involve parents in acquiring information regarding their children (See Appendix F).
- Demonstrate how to treat students with visual impairments with respect and courtesy. Speak to the class when you are entering or leaving the room as a courtesy to the student with a visual impairment. This will act as a role model for other students to follow your lead in acceptance of them.
- Introduce the student with visual impairments as you would any other student. It is not important to tell about his or her condition as the other students will ask questions in time and the student with the visual impairment will answer them himself or herself.
- Unless students with visual impairments know you well, state your name as you come upto them. Speak directly to the student and not through a third person. Call him or her by name when you want his or her attention.
- Use the words 'see' and 'look' when speaking with students with visual impairments. One should make his/her conversation as normal as possible since these students want to be treated the same as everyone else.
- Verbal cues need to be used whenever necessary. This is more so as students with visual impairments may not be ableto see and understand body language. Moreover, they may also fail to understand what it means foran object to be 'here' or 'there'.
- Every effort must be made to include students with visual impairments in all activities within the school curriculum (physical education, home economics, music). Participation in these classes and extracurricular activities provides excellent opportunities for developing leisure skills and social skills.

- Encourage students with visual impairments to take leadership roles in the same manneras you would encourage other students.
- Be aware of the amount of assistance which students with visual impairments need before offering help. You may need to encourage them to accept more help or be willing to do things more independently.
- Allow students with visual impairments to bring any required adaptive aids to class. They can also explain how these aids work to their classmates if they so desire. This will help classmates feel more comfortable with studentswith visual impairments and facilitate closer interaction.
- If a student is having a problem with a particular task, consult with the Itinerant Teacher to determine whether other adaptations are necessary or if the task is just too difficult for the student's abilities.
- The teacher needs to use same forms of discipline for students with visual impairments as for anyother student.
- Some students who are blind or visually impaired display certain mannerisms (rocking, fingers in the eyes or eye—poking, repetitive movements). Encourage him or her to lessen these mannerisms. The teacher can consult the Special Education Teacher or Itinerant Teacher regarding this.
- Realise that a student with a visual impairment tends to tire more easily than a sighted student when performing near tasks such as reading. Be prepared to offer brief breaks to the student or to change types of tasks when necessary.
- Help students develop a realistic balance between what is possible and what is practical in order to avoid feelings of frustrations.
- Consult with the Itinerant Teacher or Special Education Teacher regularly to develop ways to appropriately programme so that students with visual impairments get the maximum benefits (See Appendix G).

8

Accessibility and Infrastructure for Persons with Disabilities in India

Infrastructural development is one of the key determinants of a Nation's progress. This calls for effective planning, developing, managing and executing infrastructure in an equitable manner so that its benefit can be derived by all sections of the society including persons with disabilities (PWDs). Unfortunately, the provision of safe, accessible and affordable sustainable transport for disabled people often gets little or no attention from transport planners in developing countries due to the ignorance of the accessibility component in both formulations of policies as well as in their implementation. With these in view, the chapter aims at critically analysing the existing infrastructure elements for persons with disabilities such as accessible services and facilities and also evaluates and assesses the public transportation services as relevant in the Indian scenario.

The passage of the Persons with Disabilities (Equal Opportunities, Protection of Rights and Full Participation) Act, 1995 and India signing and ratifying the UN Convention for Protection of Rights of Disabled Persons had resulted in a few developments. Although limited but changes were evident by way of increased cooperation and coordination between the user groups, NGO's and the stakeholders as a result of infrastructural development and building and municipality bylaws. Airports and road and built infrastructure have incorporated the principles of Universal Design so as to make them more accessible by the PWDs. The Jawaharlal Nehru Urban Renewal Mission Plan attempted to introduce low floor buses in metropolitan cities-Delhi, Mumbai, Kolkata, Hyderabad, Bangalore, Chennai and any other cities with population between one million to four million. Even the Indian Railways manufactured 2,100 specially designed non-airconditioned coaches having accommodation for the disabled. Presently, A1 Class-58, A Class-284, B Class-138 stations are accessible.

In lieu of the changes, it is quite correct to state that much of the changes initiated by the government have been the result of pressure from the disability sector. This has ensured few disabled friendly buses, some accessible public places and comparatively greater awareness about the issue.

However, a comprehensive glance at the prevailing conditions glaringly points out to the need for greater and more focussed initiatives and actions by policy makers as well as implementing agencies. It becomes increasingly apparent from a close and critical view of the accessible transport services for people with disabilities that the root of the problem lies in the very perception of people with disabilities. Most people still regard disability to be a static condition rather than an interaction between an individual and a non-inclusive society. This bears severe adverse affect on the initiatives been undertaken for people with disabilities. Due to this, disability itself is regarded as a factor hindering equal participation of persons with disabilities in society, whilst the real obstacle is a resultant of overwhelming environmental barriers, including inaccessible transport systems with poor infrastructure, vehicle design and information provision.

Review of various books, articles and government and other related documents have revealed a rather dismissal picture of safe and accessible transport for people with disabilities in India.

It is rather unfortunate that although the National Urban Transport Policy dwells on all issues related to urban transport but does not address issue of accessible transport to disabled people and elderly people. Although the policy states 'accessing jobs, education, recreation and similar activities is becoming increasingly time consuming', but it overlooks that an accessible transport system can become a medium for better access to education and jobs for persons with disabilities. Even though certain legislative measures have been enacted but they are poorly enforced and rarely implemented. The Indian legislation requires that trains and buses reserve seats reserved for passengers with disabilities and that these passengers receive fare concessions, but such promising laws are rarely enforced. For instance, the city of Bangalore has low floor buses (Volvo) but the disability concession is not valid in these buses and the fare/rate is higher, making them again inaccessible for majority of people with disabilities.

Under the title 'Promotion of Non-handicapping Environment for Disabled and Elderly Persons', the Annual Report of Ministry of Urban Development proudly mentions that 'Efforts will be made to ensure adoption of Bye-laws and space standards by all states, municipal bodies, and panchayati raj institutions in the country. These authorities will ensure that all newly constructed buildings for public-use are barrier-free. Regarding accessibility and barrier-free environment, it further goes on to add that the Ministry has prepared Model Building by laws, which contain provisions for improving access to various public buildings by disabled and elderly persons. These building by-laws have been sent to the state governments, union territories, Delhi Development Authority, Municipal Corporation of Delhi, New Delhi Municipal Committee, etc., for adoption. So far, Maharashtra, Tripura, Gujarat, Meghalaya, Karnataka, Bihar, Andhra Pradesh, National Capital Territory of Delhi and Chandigarh have adopted the same. All states have been asked to appoint an officer in every district to bring to notice cases of non-compliance to the concerned authorities. However, based on the information given in the Annual Report, only nine states in India have adopted the by-laws but it fails to specify as to how these state governments have implemented them. Although the Annual Report states that an officer in each district would be appointed divulge no information regarding their appointment or the work undertaken by them.

Another major constraint is the lack of adequate understanding about what nature of accessibility is needed for people with disabilities in the country. There are no standards that are followed in the construction of ramps, washrooms and other facilities for disabled people. Accessibility provisions for persons with disabilities are merely associated and confined to mere construction of ramps which also rarely comply with the standards of construction.

Several features have been identified causing problems for pedestrians, particularly those with mobility difficulties such as unsuitable walkways, street crossings; fast and heavy traffic; high, narrow and uneven sidewalks; inaccessible subways; ramps and steps; inadequate signages; car parks and transport interchanges Hitchcock and Mitchell, 1984). Table 8.1 indicates the percentage of people with different degrees of disability who are affected by various features. It was found that although some features such as narrow or uneven sidewalks, and crossing roads affect everyone but they gravel affect people with disabilities.

Table 8.1: Percentage of People with Disabilities Affected by Various Aspects of Pedestrian Environment

Aspect of pedestrian environment	*Registered disabled*
Kerbs	12
Steps	58
Hills/ramps	59
Uneven/narrow Sidewalks	21
Crowds	50
Traffic/crossing roads	35
No difficulties	2
Sample size	143

Source: Hitchcock and Mitchell (1984).

In the survey, virtually all respondents reported having had at least one accident whilst out walking, and over half had sustained injuries. Pedestrians with vision impairment reported of experiencing higher frequencies of walking accidents and injuries than sighted people. They specified of undergoing more accidents than sighted people when crossing roads and over a third of respondents experienced accidents involving steps.

Accessible footways are often evidently absent making the roads highly unsafe for people with disabilities. Despite The Disability Act, 1995 advocating disabled-friendly roads, streets, etc. and the Annual Report or the Eleventh Plan mandating audio signals, most of the subways, foot-over bridges etc. yet remain inaccessible for people with disabilities. Groundless and hilarious initiatives have been adopted causing inevitable embarrassment such as providing whistles to visually impaired people in Bangalore in order to stop vehicles while crossing.

Road transport, i.e., buses, cars, auto rickshaws, etc., is largely inaccessible to people with disabilities. This makes it impossible for not only the orthopedically disabled but also persons with visual disability and with hearing impairment to use public buses in the country. The problems are wide ranged from the route number of the bus being not visible, inaccessible bus stops, lack of adequate communication with the conductor, lack of cooperation from the bus driver to stop the bus at the bus stop to lack of sign boards at the bus terminals, display boards or announcements for latest updates.

It is significant to consider that although a few 'disabled-friendly' buses have been introduced in a few cities in the country as a result of Public Interest Litigation (PIL) and activism but they fail to be friendly to visually impaired commuters. Most disabled people still undergo the plight of travelling in regular buses which adheres to a transport policy that does not take into account the concerns of people with disabilities.

In the shadow of providing helpful initiatives, shocking suggestions have been placed forth such as introducing special bus service for people with disabilities rather than initiating concrete efforts towards making urban transport system universally accessible to all. The concept of a special provision itself points out shamelessly to denial of the very essence of the inclusion policy.

Highlighting on the issue of ensuring greater accessibility for persons with disabilities, the Eleventh Plan stated that all mail and express trains would be provided with specially designed coaches that have separate compartments and suitably designed toilets for the physically challenged and senior citizens. In addition, trains having air-conditioned accommodation would also be provided with air-conditioned compartments for physically challenged persons. However, in reality, the placement of the disabled-friendly coaches at the either end of the train has ensured complete failure of the fundamental principle of convenience and accessibility for people with disabilities. As a consequence, these coaches are rarely occupied by its rightful owners. Moreover, lack of attendants to cater to the arising needs of the passengers, nonexistence of vestibule to move from one compartment to another, its disconnection with the pantry car have all made this provision not preferred and inaccessible by people with disabilities.

Although the NGO s have played a significant role in addressing the various issues of persons with disabilities, it is difficult to deny that the knowledge and expertise in the field of accessibility is limited even within the NGO sector. These loopholes vehemently points out to the fact that accessibility issues are neither regarded as national or state level developmental plans and nor are persons with disabilities perceived as consumers of services.

Initiatives

The main issue that arises here is whether the government proposing mere reservation of a bus or a train compartment ensures humane treatment for people with disabilities. The answer surely is NO! Significant improvements are needed in the pedestrian network. Certain focussed actions need to be undertaken by different stakeholders in improving accessibility to transportation by people with disabilities in India. Key stakeholders like the national government, city government, civil society, development agencies and the private sector need to support the development and implementation of these actions. The national government should play a substantial role especially in relation to development of national standards for pedestrian facilities and in supporting local governments in developing local action plans for improving transportation accessibility. It is imperative that the guidelines and space standards for barrier-free built environment for disabled and elderly persons, by Central Public Works Department as specified by the Ministry of Urban Affairs and Employment (1998) be put to full-fledged implementation. One needs to adhere to the specific requirements of constructing suitable walks and paths for the disabled pedestrians. The walks should be smooth, hard level surface suitable for walking and wheeling. Irregular surface as cobble stones, coarsely exposed aggregate concrete, bricks, etc., often cause bumpy rides. Longitudinal walk gradient should be three to five per cent (30 mm-50 mm in one metre) and when walks exceed 60 metre in length it is desirable to provide rest area adjacent to the walk at convenient intervals with space for bench seats. For comfort the seat should be between 350 mm-425 mm high but not over 450 mm. The texture change in walkways adjacent to seating will be desirable for blind persons.

Detailed efforts need to be made to take notice of the Signages. The main purpose of signs should be to provide a clear designation of places, warnings and routing information. Contrasting texture alongside walkways and audible signs for dangerous areas should be provided for a partially sighted person. Efforts should be made to ensure that signs should be useful to everyone, be easily seen from eye level, be readable by moving the fingers and well lighted for right time identification. Care should be taken to ensure that signs indicate the direction and name of the accessible facility and incorporate the symbol of access. The size, type and layout of lettering on signs shall be clear and legible. Signs should be in contrasting colours and preferably be embossed in distinct relief to allow visually impaired persons to obtain the information they contain by touching them. Provision of illuminated signages, layout diagrams should be provided to help people with hearing disabilities easily reach the desired place.

Besides these, one needs to ensure safe crossing facilities for persons with wheel chair and with impaired vision by providing acoustic signal and installing a safety zone on a wide road. Provision of kerb ramp needs to be provided at appropriate location at the footpath. Other provisions need to be made available in the form of guiding block at the starting and ending of crossing, accessible bus stop/taxi stand, accessible subway/overbridge, accessible concourse, ticket booth of the railway station, installation of guiding blocks on the concourse for persons with impaired vision, etc., to facilitate easy access to roadways and transportation for people with disabilities. Even an appropriate number of designated seats for passengers with disabilities need to be provided near doors.

Understanding these constraints and the urgency of overcoming them, Julie put together a table showing a continuum of necessary interventions for countries to make their transport systems accessible for all (See Table 8.2). They include adequate railings and ramps for footbridges; obstacle-free footways with ramps and tactile markings; extended lights at pedestrian crossings; and adequate signage. For public transit, they include reducing gaps between trains/buses and platforms, and ensuring that steps are low and have hand grasps.

Table 8.2: Continuum of Necessary Interventions for Countries to Make their Transport Systems Accessible for all

Infrastructure	*Women (~50% pop)*	*Children (~25-50% pop)*	*Elderly (~10-25% pop)*	*Disabled (~10-12% pop)*
Footbridges	Adequate clear width and height; railings; ramps.			
Sidewalks/ curbs	Elimination of obstacles; ramps and adequate gradients; tactile markings; signboards and signs with accessible pedestrian signals (APS); adequate lighting; longer settings for street crossing			
Train/bus stations	Platform and train gap elimination; adequate lighting; warning and signs of possible dangers			
Vehicles (buses, trains, private)	Low steps; hand grasps; good information display of destination; keeping vehicle stationary longer; priority seating			

Source: Julie Babinard, 2010.

It is also important for civil society to be involved in developing and monitoring the implementation of these policies and activities. Development agencies should play active roles in establishing and supporting initiatives for improving walking environments for people with disabilities such as supporting the development of pedestrian-related polices, reviewing design guidelines for transport and pedestrian facilities and walkability assessment standards ensuring their inclusion into the mainstream society.

Conclusion

Finally, all evidence suggests that transportation is a necessary but not a sufficient condition for the full access and mobility of travelers with disabilities. It is necessary that transportation planners must work in cooperation with both the public and the private sectors and with professionals in a variety of disciplines and service delivery systems to address the access and mobility needs of a range of travelers with disabilities. However, it needs to be borne in mind that none of these involve huge investments but they certainly do require sufficient political will and desire to initiate and execute.

9

Issues and Challenges in the Employment of Persons with Disabilities in India

The fast changing socio-economic scenario in the country and its impact on urbanisation, industrialisation and modernisation of the economy has resulted in increasing trends of rural-urban drift in search of livelihood leading to a strain on the already limited urban facilities, resulting in serious problems of over-crowding, increase in slum dwellers, unemployment, poverty, destitution, etc. All these factors have exposed the vulnerable and the disadvantaged to the increasing incidence of social deviance and maladjustment. In keeping view of this, the National Human Rights Commission (NHRC) has taken several initiatives to protect the rights of the disabled. Several legislative measures have initiated for the rehabilitation and empowerment of certain categories of disability such as, The Rehabilitation Council of India Act (1992); The National Trust For Welfare of Persons With Autism, Cerebral Palsy, Mental Retardation and Multiple Disabilities Act (1999) and Persons With Disabilities (Equal Opportunities, Protection of Rights and Full Participation) Act, 1995.

India being one among the signatories of The Convention on the Rights of Persons with Disabilities and its Optional Protocol adopted on 13 December, 2006 at the United Nations Headquarters in New York is obliged to organise, strengthen and extend comprehensive habilitation and rehabilitation services and programmes, particularly in the areas of health, employment, education and social services (Article 26). In 1997, the Government of India incorporated the National Handicapped Finance and Development Corporation (NHFDC) in order to help entrepreneurs with disabilities through financial assistance.

Besides the policies emphasising on vocational empowerment, Employment Exchanges under the National Employment Services as well as Special Employment Exchanges have been entrusted with the responsibility for the placement of persons with disabilities. These exchanges attempt to secure for the disabled the most satisfying form of employment suitable to their residual physical and mental potentialities. At present, 42 Special Exchanges are in operation. In addition to this, 41 Special Cells for disabled persons with a Special Placement Officer attached to the normal Employment Exchanges and funded by the Central Government have also been set up by the Ministry of Social Justice and Empowerment. Table 9.1 shows the performance of the Special Employment Exchange for Persons with Disabilities in 1999.

Table 9.1. Performance of the Special Employment Exchange for Persons with Disabilities in 1999

Registration	*Placement*	*Active Register*
62.7	4.2	455,900

(*Source:* Annual Report 2001-2002, Ministry of Labour, Government of India: p. 242).

Critical Review of the Policies and the Legislation Process

It is evident from the 'People with Disabilities in India: From Commitments to Outcomes' (2007) report that there has been a five per cent drop in the employment rate of people with disabilities in the decade leading up to 2002. The fall in the employment rate of working age disabled people has been from

42 per cent in 1991 to 37 per cent in 2002 (for state-wise data see Table 9.2). This makes it imperative to analyse some of the issues causing this backlog in the area of employment of people with disabilities in India.

Table 9.2: Employment Rates of Persons with Disabilities by State/ Union Territory

State	*1999-2000 Employment Rate-All India*			*2002 Employment Rate Disabled*		
Andhra Pradesh	All	Rural	Urban	All	Rural	Urban
Assam	71.52	80.10	51.69	37.89	39.19	33.66
Bihar	54.40	55.42	47.29	32.48	33.42	23.62
Gujarat	56.08	58.19	43.17	37.12	37.99	30.22
Haryana	68.29	77.36	50.57	39.28	41.50	34.96
Himachal Pradesh	55.88	59.15	48.50	39.37	39.41	39.20
Jammu and Kashmir	72.83	75.64	47.29	45.64	46.09	38.41
Karnataka	59.24	63.54	43.11	31.64	31.15	34.16
Kerala	67.87	74.21	52.49	38.00	38.70	35.70
Madhya Pradesh	54.24	55.02	52.09	30.41	30.88	28.93
Maharashtra	70.31	76.74	50.04	38.88	39.41	37.05
Manipur	65.89	76.38	50.95	42.13	45.36	35.26
Meghalaya	54.33	56.29	48.63	21.91	22.69	19.62
Nagaland	74.42	80.76	46.01	34.17	34.94	24.85
Orissa	64.02	71.63	46.90	31.20	35.82	15.61
Punjab	62.71	65.76	48.30	30.17	30.67	24.75
Rajasthan	60.19	64.68	51.53	40.15	40.90	37.95
Sikkim	69.44	75.22	51.14	40.52	41.65	36.78
Tamil Nadu	59.13	59.72	53.54	46.76	46.91	42.86
Tripura	66.47	72.44	55.80	38.18	38.63	37.23
Uttar Pradesh	46.06	46.53	43.49	29.65	28.68	33.84
West Bengal	57.82	60.22	49.16	36.33	36.37	36.13
Andaman and Nicobar	54.08	55.69	48.96	38.41	39.88	34.28
Arunachal Pradesh	56.96	56.08	59.01	44.59	43.35	50.00
Chandigarh	58.15	59.28	44.92	29.46	29.52	23.36
Dadra and Nagarhaveli	54.78	73.25	51.29	35.24	34.11	35.41

State	1999-2000 Employment Rate-All India			2002 Employment Rate Disabled		
Daman and Diu	74.49	76.91	57.20	36.25	35.37	43.18
Delhi	62.69	71.53	52.86	27.75	31.99	22.89
Goa	48.22	48.31	48.19	35.70	33.76	36.57
Lakshadweep	45.59	49.65	41.59	19.92	22.23	12.63
Mizoram	49.84	47.93	51.06	18.40	18.12	18.64
Pondicherry	69.12	78.52	55.23	30.71	32.81	27.38
N	54.79	61.37	50.51	32.16	30.56	32.99
	5,01,434	3,01,034	2,00,400	46,731	30,076	16,655

Source: NSSO Report on Disabled Persons, 58th Round, July-December 2002.

Unavailability of accurate data on status of disability in the country restricts adoption of adequate initiatives to address the needs of the disabled population. Vast difference in the estimates of disabled population as well as difference in definitions of disabilities adopted by the Census of India 2001 and National Sample Survey 58th Round has serious implications for the concerned population as it may provide incorrect direction to national policies regarding focussing the initiatives on essential issues.

One among the various factors restricting enforcement of legislative provisions for empowerment of people with disabilities has been the lack of detail follow up procedures which has been primarily left to the Court of Law. Keeping in mind the employment status of people with disabilitiesit is obvious that although it is legally mandatory only for public sector undertakings (PSU) to have over three per cent reservation for persons with disabilities in their workforce and PSUs such as BHEL, Hindustan Petroleum Corporation, Bharat Petroleum Corporation and National Thermal Power Corporation have toed the line but, they are primarily engaged in back-end jobs requiring only low-level skills. This also highlights loopholes in the legislative measures both in principle and practice with regard to requirement of specific post-identification (See Table 9.3). The list of identified jobs is very restricted, often arbitrary and based on the assumption that the characteristics of impairment are exclusive determinants of an individual's ability to hold a position at a particular skill level. This signifies the tendency of ignoring the potential influences of individual characteristics, access to employment services, and the characteristics of the workplace and labour market.

Table 9.3: Reserved Posts for PWD Identified and Filled, Early 2000s

Group of posts	*All posts*	*Posts identified for PWD*	*Employed PWD*	*% identified posts filled by PWD*	*% all posts filled by PWD*
Ministries and Departments					
A	57,643	4,305	134	3.11%	0.23%
B	73,851	4,652	205	4.41%	0.28%
C	1,607,243	167,863	6,307	3.76%	0.39%
D	960,025	104,578	3,329	3.18%	0.35%
Total	2,698	762 281	398 9,975	3.54%	0.37%
Public Establishments					
A	204,127	18,244	508	2.78%	0.25%
B	175,159	14,350	1,226	8.54%	0.70%
C	1,013,917	89,789	4,525	5.04%	0.45%
D	435,328	56,615	3,819	6.75%	0.88%
Total	1,828,531	178,998	10,078	5.63%	0.55%
All					
Total	4,527,293	460,396	20,053	4.36%	0.44%

Source: DOPT. Ministries and Departments were reported for 59 MandD in 1/2003 for posts as of 1/2000. The information on public establishments was reported for 237 public establishments in July 2002.

Another significant feature of the quota policy is that it is applicable only to three disability types – locomotor, visual and hearing with a one per cent reservation for each. This makes it evident that neither the disability categories of the Act nor the other categories of disabilities are included in the reservation policy. Hence, the public employment quota for persons with disabilities is narrow in its goal and has failed to provide adequate representation of them in the public sector workforce.

A critical view of the economic situation of disabled persons in India indicates that there are about 700,000 persons with disability registered with the employment exchanges. Out of these, 100,000 persons with disabilities have been successful in getting employment. Of these, 100,000, 90 per cent have locomotor impairments, about five per cent are hearing impaired and theremaining five per cent have visual impairments, ranging from partial vision to total blindness.It is obvious from the critical analysis of the impact of the employment exchanges for persons with disabilities, in Table 9.4 showing the number of PWD registered, being placed and mentioned on the live register of the special employment exchanges and other exchanges from 1994 through 2003, that placement ratio both in the special exchanges and other exchanges are very low, i.e., 0.9 per cent and 0.7 per cent respectively in 2003 reflecting significant fall in job opportunities in the public sector.

Table 9.4: PWD placed by employment exchanges (in thousands)

Registrations	*Placements*	*Live Register*		*Placement ratio*
Special Employment Exchanges				
1994	8.4	1.3	67.1	1.94%
1999	15.1	1.3	96.2	1.35%
2000	14.8	1	101.1	0.99%
2001	12	1.1	107.8	1.02%
2002	11.6	1	110.6	0.90%
2003	10.9	1	109.9	0.91%
Other Exchanges				
1994	35.3	3.2	273.2	1.17%
1999	47.6	2.9	359.7	0.81%
2000	49.9	2.3	384.1	0.60%
2001	48.1	2.4	402.2	0.60%
2002	47.8	2.4	422.1	0.57%
2003	55.2	3.9	551.8	0.71%

Source: GoI (2005).

Interestingly, the 1995 PWD Act also offers incentives to

employers ensuring that at least five per cent of their workforce is composed of persons with disabilities. So far, the government has not declared any sops nor the private sector has any such legal compulsions as a result of which they can choose not to hire people with disabilities. In addition to this, there is no appropriate information on the status of the implementation of the three per cent reservation in government jobs provided under the 1995 Act in the annual reports of the Chief Commissioner for Persons with Disabilities, the Ministry for Social Justice and Empowerment and the Ministry of Labour over the last four years. The Census 2001 shows that 49 per cent of the disabled population is literate and only 34 per cent are employed indicating that even government organisations have not managed to meet the three per cent job reservations for persons with disability. A 1999 survey held by the National Centre for Promotion of Employment of Disabled People (NCPEDP) in 100 major companies maintains said the average employment rate of the disabled people in the public sector was 0.54 per cent, 0.28 per cent in the private sector and a mere 0.05 per cent in multinational companies. This shows that though there has been an increase in the figures during the eight years but there is still a long way to go before the Disability Act's recommended five per cent rate of employment can be achieved. The NSSO Report on Disabled Persons, 58th Round, July-December 2002 also shows a dismissal picture concerning the employment of the disabled persons in India in the various professions and sectors as shown in Table 9.5.

Regarding promotion of self-employment among persons with disabilities, the number of NHFDC beneficiaries between 1997

Table 9.5: Distribution of Working Age Persons with Disabilities by Usual Activity Status (15 to 64 years) in 2002

	All	*Male*	*Female*	*Rural*	*Rural*		*Urban*	*Urban*		*Mental Illness*	*Mental Retardation*	*Visual*	*Hearing*	*Speech*	*Loco-motor*	*Multiple*
					Male	*Female*		*Male*	*Female*							
Employed	37.6	51.0	16.1	38.4	51.7	16.8	34.9	48.6	13.6	9.6	15.6	21.7	58.8	49.8	41.7	33.3
Self-employed as an own account worker	14.1	20.8	3.2	14.4	21.4	3.0	12.9	18.8	3.9	1.2	4.2	8.5	20.0	12.8	17.4	8.5
Self-employed as an employer	0.4	0.5	0.1	0.4	0.5	0.1	0.3	0.5	0.0	0.0	0.1	0.3	0.7	0.1	0.4	0.3
Self-employed as helper	6.5	8.1	3.9	7.5	9.2	4.7	3.1	4.3	1.4	4.2	3.7	3.5	8.7	12.2	6.5	8.4
Regular wage/ salaried employee	4.8	6.5	2.1	2.9	3.9	1.2	11.3	15.4	4.9	0.5	1.1	2.1	3.8	3.7	6.6	3.2
Casual labour in public works	0.1	0.2	0.0	0.1	0.2	0.0	0.2	0.3	0.1	0.1	0.0	0.0	0.2	0.3	0.1	0.2
Casual labour in other types of works	11.7	14.8	6.7	13.1	16.4	7.7	7.0	9.3	3.3	3.6	6.4	7.2	25.5	20.6	10.7	12.8
Unemployed	1.2	1.6	0.5	1.0	1.3	0.4	1.9	2.7	0.7	0.1	0.2	0.6	0.6	1.9	1.7	0.6
Not in labour force	61.2	47.4	83.4	60.6	47.0	82.7	63.2	48.8	85.8	90.4	84.3	77.8	40.6	48.3	56.7	66.1
Educational Institutions	6.4	7.5	4.7	5.7	7.0	3.7	8.8	9.2	8.2	2.7	1.1	3.0	2.4	8.0	9.2	3.0
Domestic duties	13.4	0.8	33.8	12.7	0.7	32.2	15.8	1.1	39.0	4.8	6.9	12.5	20.7	16.3	13.7	12.5
Domestic duties and free collection of goods	3.5	0.7	8.2	4.1	0.8	9.4	1.7	0.2	4.0	0.9	2.8	2.8	6.9	6.8	3.2	3.6
Rentiers, pensioners, remittance recipients	1.3	1.3	1.2	1.1	1.1	1.3	1.7	2.2	1.0	0.2	0.7	2.2	2.2	0.6	1.2	0.8
Not able to work owing to disability	30.2	30.9	29.0	30.6	31.2	29.6	28.8	29.9	27.1	69.7	61.9	46.0	3.9	10.7	24.7	38.7
Beggars, prostitutes	0.7	0.8	0.6	0.6	0.7	0.4	1.2	1.2	1.3	0.2	0.4	1.7	0.2	0.2	0.6	1.7
Others	5.7	5.5	6.0	5.9	5.6	6.3	5.1	5.0	5.2	11.9	11.0	9.6	4.4	5.8	4.1	5.7
Total	46,731	29,000	17,727	30,076	18,693	11,383	16,655	10,311	6,344	2,318	4,395	4,392	4,255	2,140	24,291	4,940

and 2005 has been very low, i.e., 19,643. Apart from this even the disbursements have been very low ranging between 23 and 26 per cent of available funds in 1997-2002 partly due to long lags between receipt of funds by SCAs and loan disbursement. Moreover, with nearly 80 per cent of beneficiaries being only men and nearly 90 per cent of the beneficiaries of schemes being persons with orthopaedic disabilities it is apparent that disbursement is more driven by institutional factors rather than size of disabled population, limitations in the credit markets, etc.

Apart from the above factors, it also becomes imperative to observe Section 47 (ii)) of the PWD Act which categorically mentions non-discrimination in the matter of promotion in the area of employment on the ground of disability. Even the UNCRPD prohibited any discrimination on the basis of disability with regard to all matters concerning all forms of employment, including conditions of recruitment, hiring and employment, continuance of employment, career advancement and safe and healthy working conditions. However, in operation, the recruitment rules containing medical standards to be met by a successful candidate in selection for a given post-impedes the employment of disabled persons on various occasions. For instance, the selection test for Indian Administrative Service Cadre disqualified visually disabled persons from holding posts falling in Indian Administrative Service Cadre until the aforesaid rule was struck down by the Hon'able Supreme Court of India on a petition filed by National Federation of the Blind in the year 1993. Similarly, persons with intellectual disabilities could not access various employment opportunities in open market as they are not considered a party competent to enter into a contract as per Indian Contract Act. Besides these, Section 3 of the Apprenticeship Act, 1961, by implication, debars persons with disabilities from availing of training opportunities as apprentice as it lays down that a person shall not be qualified for being engaged as an apprentice to undergo apprenticeship training in any designated trade, unless he – (a) is not less than 14 years of age and (b) satisfies such standards of education and physical fitness as may be prescribed. Thus, it precludes persons with disabilities, from their inclusion in apprenticeship training opportunities on the ground of their not meeting their set medical standards.

Suggestive Measures

In lieu of some of the loopholes in employment for people

with disabilities, efforts need to be made for making proper use of existing vocational services, guidance and training, placement in employment and related services for workers. In addition to this, there is the need to specify procedures conforming to their employment, salary standards as well as supporting and incentive measures. Besides these, there is also the need to extend provisions for formal employment, self-employment cooperatives and other group income generating schemes.

Moreover, it is imperative that the policies for promotion of training and employment of the disabled and non-disabled persons should be adopted on an equal basis including the women. There is the need to develop a strategy for initiating as well as implementing an affirmative action for their employment. The three per cent allocation of the budget needs to be reconsidered to mainstream people with disabilities into the employment scenario. This also calls for the need to strengthen the monitoring mechanisms to supervise the progress. However, the most important initiative that needs to taken is to change the mindset of the general population towards the inclusion of people with disabilities into the mainstream society as well those involved inrecruitment/ appointment process.

Conclusion

Critical analysis of all the guidelines measures laid down by the various policies reveals that although emphasis has been laid in legislative framework for promoting employment of people with disabilities, they have failed to produce a significant impact. This signifies that all the piecemeal efforts need to be replaced by more well planned and coordinated measures. It is important to provide specifications regarding the summary procedures to be adopted thereby not leaving the enforcement of the provisions to persons with disabilities solely with the court of law. There is urgent need to create awareness of schemes and persons with disabilities entitlements in the public and non-governmental sectors and to mobilise formation of Self-Help groups, intermediary organisations such as MFIs, NGOs as well as the PWD themselves, so that there is more bottom-up demand on the delivery system.

10

Rehabilitative Services

With increase in consideration of quality parametres in all spheres of life including availability, access, and provision of comprehensive services to the disabled, it is pertinent to have a look on the contribution of government in keeping the aspiration and commitment towards common people. The chapter attempts to review the concept of rehabilitation for the people with disabilities with special reference to people with visual impairment.

Traditionally rehabilitation of the visually impaired used to be institution based and provided by organisations concerned with the welfare of the blind. To acquire indepth view of the need and scope for rehabilitation for the visually impaired, it is imperative to understand the very essence of rehabilitation. Rehabilitation involves within its domain combined and coordinated use of medical, social, educational, and vocational measures for training or retraining the individual to the highest possible level of functional ability. The three main strategies for rehabilitation of disabled are institution-based, outreach and community-based.

In general, rehabilitation encompasses the following:

- Early detection, diagnosis, and intervention;

- Improve, facilitate, stimulate and/or provide services for people with .disabilities, their families and attendant;
- Medical rehabilitation, i.e., management of curable disability and lessening the disability to the extent possible;
- Social, psychological, and other types of counseling and assistance;
- Training in self-care activities including social graces, etiquette, mobility, communication, and daily living skills with special provisions as needed;
- Provision of technical, mobility and other devices;
- Specialised education services;
- Vocational rehabilitation services including vocational guidance, training, open placement, and self-employment;
- Certification of degree of disability and provision of available concessions/benefits;
- Community awareness, advocacy, empowerment; and
- Follow-up.

The Constitution of India ensures equality, freedom, justice, and dignity of all individuals and implicitly mandates an inclusive society for all including persons with disabilities (PWDs). This necessitates the need to maintain balance between individual autonomy and community protection. Formulation of various legislation and policies play a dominant role in achieving the fundamental goals of protection, promotion and growth of individuals, groups and vulnerable population. In the recent years, there have been vast and positive changes in the perception of the society towards PWDs. It has been realised that provision of equal opportunities and effective access to rehabilitation measures can ensure better quality of life for majority of PWDs. In keeping with this objective, the Government of India has undertaken various legislative measures. It has enacted three legislations for PWDs (Refer to Appendix H, I and J for details), namely,

- National Trust for Welfare of Persons with Autism, Cerebral Palsy, Mental Retardation and Multiple Disability Act, 1999.

- Persons with Disability (Equal Opportunities, Protection of Rights and Full Participation) Act, 1995.
- Rehabilitation Council of India Act, 1992.

Seven national levels institutes have been set up to cater to the diverse needs of people with disabilities, viz,

- National Institute for the Visually Handicapped, Dehradun;
- Ali Yavar Jung National Institute for the Hearing Handicapped (AYJNIHH), formerly known as National Institute for the Hearing Handicapped, Mumbai;
- National Institute for the Mentally Handicapped, Secunderabad;
- National Institute for the Orthopedically Handicapped, Kolkata;
- National Institute of Rehabilitation Training and Research, Cuttack;
- Institute for the Physically Handicapped, New Delhi;
- National Institute for the Empowerment with Persons with Multiple Disabilities, Chennai.

National Institute for the Visually Handicapped, Dehradun

The institute, located in Dehradun, was established in 1979 by upgrading the National Centre for the Blind. It was registered as a society in 1982 under Societies Registration Act, 1860, under the administrative control of the Ministry of Social Justice and Empowerment. The institute has its regional centre in Chennai to provide rehabilitation services in the southern states of the country. It renders vocational training at par with NIVH. It also provides rehabilitation services to the rural-based visually handicapped persons through its community based rehabilitation activities. It renders services such as vocational training, manpower development, research and development, crisis management including therapeutic assistance, placement and employment, production of reading material, manufacture of aids and appliances, and library and information services, education for the visually handicapped.

The institute has a Model School for the Visually Handicapped which provides education to blind, partially sighted and low-vision children from Nursery to Class X. The blind children are taught through Braille and tactile sensation whereas the partially sighted and low vision children make use of magnifying devices to read the printed text. The scholars are provided with free board, lodging, clothing, tuition and other facilities besides monthly pocket money.

The institute also conducts long-term as well as short term training programmes for various professionals engaged in the service for the blind. It also conducts training courses for secondary school teachers of the visually handicapped at its campus, the Blind Relief Association, New Delhi and the Blind Boy's Academy, Narendrapur, West Bengal and State Level Training Course for Primary School Teachers of the Visually Handicapped. Various aids and appliances like Braille slate, Taylor Frame, Abacus, Stylus, Chess Board, Playing Cards, Pocket Frame, Folding Stick, Braille Scale, Geo Boards, Diagram Boards, Braille Shorthand Machine, etc., are also manufactured at NIVH.

Ali Yavar Jung National Institute for the Hearing Handicapped (AYJNIHH)

Ali Yavar Jung National Institute for the Hearing Handicapped (AYJNIHH) formerly known as National Institute for the Hearing Handicapped, Mumbai was established on 9th August 1983. It is an autonomous organisation under the Ministry of Social Justice and Empowerment, Government of India, New Delhi. Regional centres of the institute have been established at Kolkata (1984), New Delhi (1986), Secundarabad (1986) and Bhubaneshwar (1986, in association with Government of Orissa). These are centres aimed at meeting the local and regional needs in terms of manpower development and services.

The District Disability Rehabilitation Centre (DDRCs) under Gramin Punarvasan Yojana (GPY), a programme of the Ministry of Social Justice and Empowerment, Government of India, was started in the year 2000. The objective of the programme is to provide total rehabilitation to persons with sensory (hearing and vision), physical and mental disabilities. Under this programme, 24 DDRCs were allotted to AYJNIHH. All the 24 DDRCs, on completion of successful establishment and running for three years, are handed over to state governments/district administration/NGO.

Composite Regional Centre (CRC), Bhopal is a service model initiated by the Ministry of Social Justice and Empowerment, Government of India, established on 14th August, 2000. The centre is functioning under the administrative control of AYJNIHH since February, 2006. One more CRC at Ahmedabad, Gujarat was established on 16th Aug, 2011 and this CRC also functioning under the administrative control of AYJNIHH.

Objectives of the Institute

- *Manpower Development:* To deal with the various aspects of rehabilitation of the hearing handicapped, various undergraduate and post-graduate courses are being offered. The institute is rated excellent by the RCI.

- *Research:* Research in the areas of identification, intervention, educational approaches, remedial teaching methods, jobs for the hearing handicapped and technology development have been carried out.

- *Educational Programmes:* By studying the existing school for the deaf, curriculum followed, methods of teaching etc. and supplementing or strengthening them by way of improving existing educational facilities and developing new strategies wherever required, newer measures such as open school for the illiterate/drop out is being conducted as model activity.

- *Service Facilities:* Strategies for early identification and rehabilitative procedures. Films and audio visuals on vocational training and job placement, etc., are being developed.

- *Community Programme:* Identification and intervention, home bound training; correspondence training and also tele-rehabilitation services are being rendered and evolved with emerging needs.

- *Material Development:* Required for (a) education, like teaching aids, audio-visuals, etc. (b) public awareness and community education, literacy programme for adult deaf, parent counselling and programme for strengthening voluntary organisations.

• *Information and Documentation*: Documenting and disseminating the latest information and developments in the science of hearing, speech and related technology is being done.

National Institute for the Mentally Handicapped, Secunderabad

The institute was registered in 1984 under Societies Registration Act, 1860 as an autonomous body under the Ministry of Social Justice and Empowerment, Government of India. The National Institute for the Mentally Handicapped (NIMH) located in Secunderabad, Andhra Pradesh, is committed to develop models of care for persons with mentally handicap, conduct research in the area of mental handicap, promote human resource development and work with mentally handicapped persons in the country. The institute has certain objectives in view:

- Develop appropriate models of care and rehabilitation for the mentally retarded persons appropriate to Indian conditions.
- Develop manpower for delivery of services to the mentally handicapped.
- Identify, conduct and coordinate research in the area of mentally handicapped.
- Provide consultancy services to voluntary organisations in the area of mentally handicapped and to assist them wherever necessary.
- Serve as a documentation and information centre in the area of mental retardation.
- Acquire relevant data to assess the magnitude/causes, rural-urban composition, socio-economic factors, etc., of mental retardation in the country.
- Promote and stimulate growth of various kinds of quality sources in the country for persons with mental retardation throughout the country.

The headquarters of the institute is based at Secunderabad, Andhra Pradesh. The Regional Centres of NIMH are located at Mumbai, Calcutta and New Delhi.

NIMH conducts various human resource development programmes such as Diploma in Mental Retardation, Degree in Mental Retardation, Diploma in Vocational Training and Employment, refresher courses, short-term courses, research and development projects etc.

National Institute for the Orthopaedically Handicapped (NIOH), Kolkata

National Institute for the Orthopaedically Handicapped was established in Calcutta in 1978 taking over from the Government of West Bengal the land and building of the erstwhile Kumar P.N. Roy Group of Hospitals. It was registered as an autonomous body in April 1982 under the Societies Registration Act, 1860.

The main objectives of the institute are to undertake manpower development, to provide services to the orthopaedically handicapped, to develop model services for the orthopaedically handicapped, to conduct and sponsor research and to provide rehabilitation services to the orthopaedically handicapped.

NIOH conducts various manpower development programmes, short courses for in-service, doctors, therapists, orthotists, prosthetists, social workers, psychologists, vocational counsellors and nurses, provides services for persons with locomotor disability for rehabilitation such as assessment, physiotherapy, occupational therapy, restorative surgery, orthotic and prosthetic, vocational counselling, etc.

National Institute of Rehabilitation Training and Research, Cuttack

Swami Vivekananda National Institute of Rehabilitation Training and Research (S.V. NIRTAR) formerly known as National Institute of Rehabilitation Training and Research, Cuttack is an autonomous institute in the field of rehabilitation functioning under the Ministry of Social Justice and Empowerment of India. The institute was conceived to provide manpower to the Artificial Limbs Manufacturing Corporation of India and created in the name of Directorate of Artificial Limbs Fitting Centre (DALFC) in March 1974 and started functioning at Safdarjung Hospital, New Delhi.

The institute conducts various courses and services such as Bachelor in Physiotherapy (B.P.T.), Bachelor in Occupational Therapy (B.O.T.), Bachelor in Prosthetics and Orthotics (BPO), Masters in Occupational Therapy (Neurology, Hand Therapy, Developmental Disabilities and Rehabilitation) and Physiotherapy (Neurology, Paediatric, Musculoskeletal and Rehabilitation) and Diplomate in National Board of Examination (DNB). It also conducts short orientation courses, continuing medical education courses for rehabilitation professionals, awareness programmes for the functionaries of government and non-government persons with disabilities and their relatives, etc.

The institute also undertakes programmes of rehabilitation and provides services to orthopaedically handicapped and allied health problems. Patients with locomotor/orthopaedic disabilities due to ailments like poliomyelitis, cerebral palsy, congenital deformities, leprosy, burn contracture, paraplegia, hemiplegia, etc., and hearing and speech disabilities are treated and rehabilitated. People with disabilities requiring artificial limbs and other rehabilitation aids and appliances are provided to prevent the impairment leading to disability and to make them near normal and to carry on their activities for daily living.

Institute for the Physically Handicapped, New Delhi

The Institute for the Physically Handicapped (IPH), located in New Delhi, functions under the administrative and financial control of the Ministry of Social Justice and Empowerment, Government of India. The institute was set up on 12th November, 1976 under the Societies Registration Act, 1860.

The main aims and objectives of the Institute are to develop manpower in the field of rehabilitation and also to serve the orthopedically handicapped of all age groups. To achieve the main objective of developing manpower of rehabilitation personnel, the institute conducts various courses such as B.Sc. (Hons) in Physiotherapy, B.Sc. (Hons) in Occupational Therapy,

B.Sc. (Hons) Physical Therapy, B.Sc. (Hons), Occupational Therapy and Diploma Course in Prosthetic and Orthotic Engineering. The institute also runs outpatient services for persons with disabilities like paraplegia, hemiplegia, arthritis, cerebral palsy, post-polio residual paralysis, congenital anomalies, etc.

National Institute for empowerment of Persons with Multiple Disabilities, Chennai

National Institute for empowerment of Persons with Multiple Disabilities (NIEPMD) established in the year 2005 in Chennai under the Department of Disability Affairs, Ministry of Social Justice and Empowerment, Government of India, to serve as a national resource centre for empowerment of persons with multiple disabilities such as those with two or more disabilities in a person. The disabilities enumerated as per PWD Act, (1995) are Low Vision, Blindness, Locomotor Disability, Hearing Impairment, Mental Retardation, Mental Illness, Leprosy Cured Persons and as per The National Trust (1999) Act, are Cerebral Palsy and Autism.

The institute has certain objectives in view:

- To undertake development of human resources for management, training rehabilitation, education, employment and social development of persons with multiple disabilities.
- To promote and conduct research in all areas relating to multiple disabilities.
- To develop transdisciplinary models and strategies for social rehabilitation and to meet the needs of diverse groups of people with multiple disabilities.
- To undertake services and outreach programmes for the persons with multiple disabilities.
- The persons with multiple disabilities have equal rights to lead a better quality of life. This may be enabled with committed professionalism, accessible environment, equal opportunities, positive attitudes and appropriate, affordable, acceptable and available technological interventions.

- To provide need based comprehensive rehabilitation through team approach facilitating inclusion, ensuring empowerment of persons with multiple disabilities and their families and by substantiating field based research and development of human resources.
- Promoting quality of life for persons with multiple disabilities through equal participation of clients, families, professionals and community agencies.

It conducts long term courses such as graduate and post—graduate courses in developmental therapy, B.Ed./M.Ed. (Multiple Disabilities, PG Diploma in Early Intervention for Children with Multiple Disabilities, Diploma in Special. Education (Multiple Disabilities) and Diploma in Community Based Rehabilitation. Besides these, various short-term courses planned for medical doctors, health personnel, mobility instructors, other rehabilitation professionals and personnel, etc.

Welfare Programmes or Schemes for the Rehabilitation of People with Disabilities in India

The allocation of work related to medical component, i.e., preventative, promotive, curative aspect is primarily planned, organised, and implemented by the Union Ministry of Health and Family Welfare. Most of the rehabilitative services are rendered by the nodal agency Union Ministry of Social Justice and Empowerment and administered by states/union territories (UTs) through a number of stakeholders including ministries and department of Central/State Governments/UTs, panchayati raj institutions (PRIs), Non-governmental organisations (NGOs), disabled people organisations, advocacy groups, family and legal associations, experts and professionals for the welfare of disabled persons in the country. Some of the programmes/schemes as proposed in Union Ministry of Social Justice and Empowerment are as follows:

Schemes for National Scholarship of Persons with Disabilities

Every year 500 new scholarship are awarded for pursuing post-matric professional and technical courses of atleast one year duration under the scheme of national scholarship for PWDs.

However, scholarship are awarded for pursuing studies from IX standard onwards to students with cerebral palsy, mental retardation, multiple disabilities and profound or severe hearing impairment, students with 40 per cent or more disability whose monthly family income does not exceed Rs 15,000 are eligible for scholarship. A scholarship of Rs 700 per month to day-scholars and Rs 1,000 per month to hostlers is provided to the students pursuing graduate and post-graduate level technical or professional courses. A scholarship of Rs 400 and Rs 700 per month to hostlers is provided for pursuing diploma and certificate level professional courses. In addition to the scholarship, the students are reimbursed the course fee subject to a ceiling of Rs 10,000 per year.

National Awards for the Welfare of Persons with Disabilities

The national awards are conferred not only to individuals and organisations that are working for the welfare of the PWDs but also on PWDs having outstanding achievements. The awards are given away on 3rd December every year, which has been declared as International Day of Disabled Persons.

Deen Dayal Disabled Rehabilitation Scheme

The scheme provides support to the NGOs to deliver various rehabilitation services to people with disabilities. This includes support to schools for children with orthopedic, speech, hearing, visual and mental disabilities; vocational training centres to provide basic skills to PWDs; community-based rehabilitation program; half-way homes for psychosocial rehabilitation of treated and controlled mentally ill people; pre-school and early intervention programs; human resource development; support for setting up Braille presses; and placement services.

Scheme of Assistance to Disabled Persons for Purchase/Fitting of Aids/Appliances (ADIP Scheme)

The objective of this scheme is to assist the needy physically handicapped people with durable, modern and standard aids and appliances.

National Handicapped Finance and Development Corporation

Economic empowerment of disable persons is promoted for self-employment ventures, extend loans to PWDs for upgradation of their entrepreneurial skill, pursuing professional/technical education, and to assist self-employed individuals with disabilities in marketing their finished goods.

Science and Technology Project in Mission Mode

This project is engaged in development of technology which ultimately leads to a suitable device which is of high quality, durable, comfortable, and integrates the disabled into the mainstream of society. Funding is made available to established research and development centres, academic institutions, public sector industries, agencies undertaking research activities for the benefit of PWDs.

Various Concessions offered by the Government of India to Blind Persons

According to guidelines by the Ministry of Social Justice and Empowerment, GoI, the minimum degree of disability should be 40 per cent for an individual to be eligible for any concessions or benefits. State government also extends various benefits in addition to those initiated by the GoI.

Travel

The blind person traveling alone or with an escort on production of a certificate from a government doctor or a registered medical practitioner is eligible to get a concession to the tune of 75 per cent if traveling in first, second or sleeper class in Indian railways. The Indian Airlines Corporation allows 50 per cent concessional fare to blind persons on single journey or single fare round trip journey on all domestic flights. Escorts are to pay full fare however an air hostess/steward will look after the blind person not accompanied by escorts in flight.

Conveyance Allowances

All central government employees who are in a regular establishment and who are blind or orthopaedically handicap are to be granted conveyance allowance at five per cent of the basic pay subject to a maximum of Rs. 100 per month

Telecommunication

The blind person is entitled for rental rebate of 50 per cent on telephone facility on Non-OYT [s] category only. An educated unemployed handicap person with atleast VIIIth or middle schools pass for rural areas and matriculation or high school for urban areas is eligible for allotment of STD/PCO on priority basis

Postage

There are no postal charges levied on transmission of blind literature packets [papers, periodicals, books printed in Braille, sound records, disc films, tapes and wires for the use of the blind and when sent by, or addressed to, an officially recognised institution for the blind] to inland/foreign destination if sent by surface route weighing upto seven kg only. If packets are to be sent by air, prescribed airmail charges needs to be paid.

Concessions for Custom

Selected goods when imported into India by a disable person for their personal use are exempted from customs duty if a certificate from a government medical officer/institution certifies that import of goods is essential to overcome the said disability.

Income Tax Concessions

Section 80 DD Central Income Tax Act provides for a deduction in respect of the expenditure incurred by an individual or Hindu Undivided Family (HUF) resident in India on the medical treatment [including nursing], training and rehabilitation of handicapped dependants. Section 88 B provides for an additional rebate from net tax payable by a resident individual who has attained the age of 65 years.

Employment

Three per cent of vacancies in government employment in Grade C and D post are reserved for people with disabilities, one per cent each for persons suffering from blindness or low vision, hearing impairment and locomotor disability and cerebral palsy. The GoI has set up 47 special employment exchanges in different states for the visually handicapped. As per the decision of the GoI, it has been instructed that re-canning of chairs in government offices should be done by a visually impaired person as far as possible when the volume of work requires a full time chair caner.

Under the scheme of public sector banks for orphanages, women's homes and physically handicapped persons including blind the benefits of the differential rate of interest are available to physically handicapped persons as well as institutions working for the welfare of the handicapped. Under the integrated rural development programme (IRDP), three per cent quota is earmarked for physically handicapped persons.

Children Education Allowances

Grant of children educational allowances, reimbursement of tuition fees to central government employees are governed by central civil services order.

Scheme of Integrated Education for Disabled Children

This is centrally sponsored scheme and was launched in 1974 by the then Department of Social welfare. This scheme has, however, been transferred to the Department of Education since 1982. Under the scheme, handicapped children are sought to be integrated in the normal school system. Financial assistance to the tune of 100 per cent is provided to states/UTs for education of children suffering from certain mild handicaps in common schools with the help of necessary aids, incentives and specially trained teachers. The following types of disabled children are covered under this scheme: (a) children with locomotor handicaps; (b) mildly and moderately hearing impaired; (c) partially sighted children; (d) mentally handicapped educable group (IQ 50-70); (e) children with multiple handicap; (f) children with learning disabilities.

11

Conclusion

Critical Reflections: Concluding Thoughts and Future Possibilities

Globally, there is a conscious shift away from special schooling to mainstream schooling of education for children with disabilities. In keeping view of this, it should be our objective to make mainstream education not just available but accessible, affordable and appropriate for students with disabilities. It is true that by making our schools accessible to children with disabilities, we will also be able to improve the quality of education for all children which is a key objective of the Sarva Shiksha Abhiyan.

At the very outset, it is important to review implementation of existing programmes, provisions to identify factors leading to success or failure of the drive towards enrollment and retention of children with disabilities in mainstream educational settings.

Accessibility to educational institutions remains to be a major hurdle for students with disabilities. Thus, it is necessary to adopt precautionary measures to ensure physical access for children and youth with disabilities in schools and educational institutions to a barrier, free environment by enforcing the requirement for provisions of universal design in buildings and provide support in transportation. Supporting the entire process of inclusive education also requires the need to address issues of curriculum and pedagogy. It is significant to mention here that institutions such as the NCERT are addressing this issue and has set up a group under the National Curriculum Framework Review (2000) to examine the pedagogic inputs and classroom reorganisation required for the education of Children With Special Needs.

There is also the need to put in place an effective communication and delivery system for specific delivery of teaching/ learning material, aids and appliances, hardware/ software to the students with disabilities.

It will be possible to successfully implement integrated educational programmes only when the regular school educators are trained at a mass scale. There is the inevitable need for designing some innovative models to train teachers and equip them using unconventional training methods. In keeping view of the enormous diversity (socio-economic, linguistic, etc.) in India great care must be taken in identification of specific content to be included in the training programmes. The curriculum for pre-service training programmes need to be carefully designed based on basic skills, professional knowledge, communication and interaction skills, knowledge about assessment techniques, resource management, etc. Provisions need to be made for appropriate resource services support through appointment of special educators, rehabilitation professionals, provision of resource room, etc. to support mainstream schoolteachers in the classrooms.

There should be appropriate mechanisms to ensure a system of regular feedback and monitoring. The government clearly needs to do more than just enact legislation and announce action plans. It must put enforcing and monitoring mechanisms in place. An Action Plan for making education disabled friendly by 2020, announced by the Human Resources Development Ministry in March 2005, sets no interim targets. There is the need for greater and more focussed collaboration among the different administrative units for streamlining efforts towards effective implementation of the integrated educational programme.

While NGOs continue to be sole players in the delivery of special education through grants-in-aids received from the government their involvement needs to be actively sought in efforts toward changing the role of special education centres and meeting the goals of mainstreaming. Thus, there is a need and growing urgency to examine the role, purpose and quality of provision offered by these organisations.

Generating awareness in the general community, persons in the education field and more specifically among parents and children with disability that the disabled have full rights to appropriate education in mainstream schools and that it is the duty of those involved in administration at every level including schools to ensure that they have access to education definitely forms the most important area that needs immediate notice.

Govinda and Bandyopadhyay (2008) in their country level analysis of elementary education note that certain states have taken steps to identify children with disabilities and provide for them in regular schools there is considerable variation in efforts. For instance, Himachal Pradesh began a push towards IE in 1999-2000. A total of 25,476 children have been identified as CWSN which is 2.34 per cent of the total school going population at elementary level. At present, 23,011 of these have been integrated in mainstream schools and those out of school (2,465) are being brought into the system using different strategies, such as alternative schooling, etc. Similarly, the states of Andhra Pradesh and Orissa have also given high priority to the integration of CWSN into regular schools. Most of these piecemeal efforts have significantly pointed out to the imperative need to move beyond redistribution to reorganisation. The current approaches which are largely directed towards identification of more children, transforming special schools into resource centres, or even shifting children to mainstream settings, are inadequate. The focuss needs to shift from the outside to the 'inside'—we need to be concerned about what children are being offered in these educational settings and its relevance to the lives they would like to lead.

However, whatever and whichever be the initiatives undertaken it is important for us to raise a few very pertinent questions and seek the answers to them as early as possible. Are mere launching various schemes and programmes enough for the development of children with disabilities? Does the educational system in actual terms cater to their needs and problems or are they mere attempts towards the attainment of target goals for the proposed plans and policies? Are children with disabilities actually benefitting from the educational programmes. Is the quality of education being imported as important as the numbers enrolled? Are we really sensitised towards children with disabilities?

Bibliography

Abberley, P. (1987). The concept of oppression and the development of a social theory of disability, *Disability, Handicap, and Society*, 2, 1, 5–19.

Abner, G, and Lahm, E. (2002). Implementation of assistive technology with students who are visually impaired: Teachers' readiness. Journal of Visual Impairment and Blindness, 96, 98-105.

Bailey, J. (1998). Medical and Psychological Models in Special Needs Education.In C. Clark and A. Millwood, *Theorising Special Education*. London: Routledge.

Baine, D. (1986). *Testing and Teaching Handicapped Children and Youth in Developing Countries*. UNESCO.

Baine, D. (1988). *Handicapped Children in Developing Countries: Assessment, Curriculum and Instruction*. Edmonton: Vector Press.

Baker, K., and Donelly, M. (2001). The Social Experiences of Children with disability and the influence of environment: A framework for intervention. *Disability and Society*, 16, 1, 71-85.

Banerjee, G. (2004). *Legal Rights of Persons with Disabilities*. New Delhi: Rehabilitation Council of India.

Barnes, C. (1991). *Disabled People in Britain and Discrimination: A case for anti-discrimination legislation*. London: Hurst and Co.

Barnes, C. (1999, December). *A Working Social Model? Disability and Work in the 21st Century*. Paper Presented at the Disability Studies Conference and Seminar, Apex International Hotel, Edinburgh.

Barton, L., and Tomlinson, S. (1984). *Special Education and Social Interests*. London: Cromwell Publishers.

Battle, P., and Blowers, K. (1982). A longitudinal comparative study of the self-esteem of students in regular and special education classes.*Psychological Abstracts*, 61, 1, 233.

Bayliss, P. (1995). Segregation, integration, exclusion, inclusion: Frameworks and rationales. *Special Education Gent*, 7, 4-26.

Bear, G. G., Proctor, W. A., and Waldron, N. L. (1991). Evaluation Report: Integrating Students with Disabilities in the Least Restrictive Environment in Responses to Questions Teachers and Administrators Frequently Ask About Inclusive School Programmes. *Phi Delta Kappan*, 78, 2 150-157.

Bennett, N. (1991). The quality of classroom learning experiences for children with special educational needs. In M. Ainscow (Ed.), *Effective Schools for All*. London: David Fulton.

Bharadwaj, P. (1995). Personality factors among handicapped and non-handicapped. In M.B. Buch, *Sixth All India Educational Survey, Vol. 2*. Delhi: NCERT.

Biklen, D., Ferguson, D., and Ford, A. (1989). *Schooling and Disability II*.University of Chicago Press.

Bishop, V. (1986). Identifying the components of success in the mainstream.*Journal of Visual Impairment and Blindness*, 80, 939-946.

Blackhurst, A. E., and Berdine, W. H. (1993). *An Introduction to Special Education* (3rd ed.). New York: Harper Collins College Publishers.

Booth, T. (1991). Integration, disability and commitment: a response to Marten Soder. *European Journal of Special Needs Education*, 6, 1, 1-15.

Brinker, R. P., and Thorpe, M. E. (1985). Integration of severely handicapped students and the proportion of IEP objectives achieved. *Psychological Abstracts*, 72, 3, 886.

Bronfenbrenner, U (1989). Ecological systems theory. *Annals of Child Development*, 6, 189-249.

Bronfenbrenner, U. (1979). *The Ecology of Human development*. MA: Harvard University Press.

Bronfenbrenner, U. (1986). Ecology of the family as a context for human development: Research perspectives. *Developmental Psychology*, 22, 723-742.

Buch, M. B. (1988). *Sixth All India Educational Survey Vol. 2*. Delhi: NCERT.

Burgdorf RL, editor. The legal rights of handicapped persons: cases, materials and texts. Baltimore, MD: Paul H Brookes, 1980.

Butler, J. (1993). *Bodies that Matter: on the Discursive Limits of Sex.* London: Routledge

Byrd, E., Byrd, P.D., and Allen, C.M. (1977).Television programming and disability.*Journal of Applied Rehabilitation Counseling,* 8, 1, 28-32.

Cage, B.N. (1984). Educational Changes for the 1990s, *Phi Delta Kappan,* 20, 4, 123.

Camilleri, J.M. (1999). Disability: A Personal Odyssey. *Disability and Society,* 14, 5.

Chadwick, A. (1996). Knowledge, power and the Disability discrimination Bill.*Disability and Society,* 11, 25-40.

Christensen, C. (1993). Deviant, disabled or different: the politics of labelling. *Australian Disability Review,* 3, 5-12.

Connors, J.L., and Donnellan, A. M. (1993). Citizenship and culture: the role of disabled people in Navajo society. *Disability, Handicap and Society,* 8, 256-280.

Dash, M. (2000). *Education of Exceptional Children.* New Delhi: Atlantic Publishers.

Dawn, R. (2013). 'Education of persons with disabilities in India: A reality or a parable' in International Journal of Disability and Human Development, 12(1): 5–13.

Dawn, R. (2013). Assistive technology for Students with Visual Impairments: A Path Revisited. *Indian Educational Review*

Dawn, R. (2013). Education of Children with Disabilities in India: A Critique. *Economic and Political Weekly.*

Degerner, T., and Koster-Dreese, Y. (eds.). (1995). Human Rights and Disabled Persons: Essays and Relevant Human Rights Instruments. In G.N. Karna, *United Nations and Rights of Disabled Persons: A Study in Indian Perspective.* New Delhi: A.P.H. Publishing Corporation.

Dewsbury, G., Clarke, K., Randall, D., Rouncefield, M., and Sommerville, I. (2004).The anti-social model of disability.*Disability and Society,* 19, 2, 145-158.

Dillon, C., Byrd, K., and Byrd, D. (1980). Television and Disability. *Journal of Rehabilitation,* 46, 4, 67-69.

Donoghue, C. (2003). Challenging the Authority of the Medical Definition of Disability: an analysis of the resistance to the social constructionist paradigm. *Disability and Society,* 18, 2, 199-208.

Dowling, M., and Dolan, L. (2001). Families with Children with Disabilities—Inequalities and the Social Model. *Disability and Society*, 16, 1, 21-35.

Eccles, J., and Wigfield, A. (1985). Teacher expectations and student motivation, In J. Dusek (ed.), *Teacher expectations*. NJ: Lawrence Erlbaum.

Edwards, B. J, and Lewis, S. (1998). The use of technology in programs for students with visual impairments in Florida. *Journal of Visual Impairment and Blindness*, 92, 302-312.

Fazelhoy, R. S. (1989). Integrated Education in India: Benefits and Problems. *Journal of Visual Impairment and Blindness*, 83, 1, 47-50.

Festinger, L. (1954). A Theory of Social comparison processes. *Human Relations*, 7, 117-140.

Fine, M., and Asch, A. (1988). Disability Beyond Stigma: Social Interaction, Discrimination, and Activism. *Journal of Social Issues*, 44, 1, 3-21.

Finkelstein, V. (1990). Disability: An Administrative Challenge? In M. Oliver, *Social Work: Disabling People and Disabling Environments*. London: Jessica Kingsley Publisher.

Finkelstein, V. (1997). Emancipating Disabling Studies. In T. Shakespeare (Ed.), *The Disability Reader: Social Sciences Perspectives*. London: Cassell.

Finkelstein, V. (1998, June). *The Biodynamics of Disablement? Disability and Rehabilitation Systems Research*. Paper presented at Harare, Zimbabwe.

Finkelstein, V. (2001, December). *The Social Model of Disability Repossessed*. Paper presented at Manchaster Coalition of Disabled People.French, S. (1993). 'Can You See the Rainbow? The Roots of Denial', In J. Swain, V. Finkelstein, S. French and M. Oliver, *Disability Barriers, Enabling Environment*, Milton Keynes, U.K: Open University Press.

Foucault, M. (1972). *The Archaeology of Knowledge*. New York: Pantheon.

Foucault, M. (1973). *The Birth of the Clinic*, London: Tavistock.

French, S. (1999). 'The Wind Gets in My Way', In M. Corker and S. French (eds.), *Disability Discourse*, Milton Keynes, U.K: Open University Press.

Gartner, A., and Lipsky, D. K. (1987). Beyond Special Education: toward a quality system for all students. *Harvard Educational Review*, 57, 43, 367-395.

Ghai, A. (2000). Towards Understanding Disability. *Psychological Studies*, 45, 3, 145-149.

Gilson, S. F., and Depoy, E. (2000). Multiculturalism and Disability: A critical perspective. *Disability and Society*, 15, 2, 207-218.

Goffman, E. (1963). *Stigma: Notes on the Management of a Spoiled Identity*. New York: Simon and Schuster.

Gottlieb, J. (1981). Mainstreaming: fulfilling the promise? *American Journal of Mental Deficiency*, 86, 115-126.

Government of India (1964). *Education and National Development: Report of the Education Commission 1964-66*. New Delhi: Ministry of Human Resource Development.

Government of India (1990). *Towards an Enlightened and Humane Society: National Policy of Education, 1986-A Review Part 1*. New Delhi.

Government of India (1992). *National Policy on Education 1986: With Modifications Undertaken in 1992*. New Delhi: Ministry of Human Resource Development.

Government of India (1992). *Scheme of Integrated Education for the Disabled Children*. New Delhi: Ministry of Human Resource Development.

Government of India (1995). *The Persons With Disabilities (Equal Opportunities, Protection of Rights and Full Participation) Act, 1995*. New Delhi: Ministry of Human Resource Development.

Government of India (1995). *The Rehabilitation Council of India Act: Act No.34*. New Delhi: Ministry of Welfare.

Government of India. National Sample Survey Organisation. 58th Round. New Delhi: Ministry of Statistics and Programme Implementation, 2002.

Hahn, H. (1982). The Politics of Physical Differences: Disability and Discrimination. *Journal of Social Issues*, 44, 1, 39-47.

Hales, G. (1996). Beyond Disability: Towards Enabling Society. New Delhi: Sage Publishers.

Hallahan, D.P., and Kauffman, J.M. (1978). *Exceptional Children: Introduction to Special Education*. Englewood Cliffs, N.J: Prentice-Hall Inc. *Handicap and Society*, 4, 3, 221-239.

Harvey, D.H. (1985). Mainstreaming: Teachers' attitudes when they have no choice about the matter. *Psychological Abstract*, 73, 9, 2491.

Havill, S. (1970). The sociometric status of visually handicapped students in public schools. In M. Hoben. and V. Lindstrom, *Evidence of Isolation in the Mainstream. Journal of Visual Impairment and Blindness*, 74, 8, 289-292.

Hegarty, S., and Alur, M. (2002). *Education with Children with Special Needs: From Segregation to Inclusion*. New Delhi: Sage.

Hegarty, S., Pocklington, K., and Lucas, D. (1982). Integration in Action. In P. Bayliss, Segregation, integration, exclusion, inclusion: Frameworks and rationales. *Special Education Gent*, 7, 4-26.

Helldin, R. (2000). Special Education Knowledge Seen as a Social Problem. *Disability and Society*, 15, 2, 247-270.

Hewett, F. M., and Forness, S. R. (1984). *Education of Exceptional Learners*. Massachussetts: Allyn and Bacon Inc.

Hoben, M. (1980). Toward integration in the mainstream. *Exceptional Children*, 47, 2, 100-105.

Hoben, M., and Lindstrom, V. (1980). Evidence of Isolation in the Mainstream. *Journal of Visual Impairment and Blindness*, 74, 8, 289-292.

Howell, K. (1976). *Inside Special Education*. New York: Charles. E. Merill Co.

Hughes, H. M., and Paterson, M. (1997). The Social Model of Disability and Disappearing Body: towards a social model of impairment. *Disability and Society*, 12, 3, 325-340.

Hurt, J. (1988). *Outside the Mainstream: A history of special education*. London: Batsford.

Husain, M. G. (1984). *Problems and Potentials of the Handicapped*. New Delhi: Atlantic Publishers.

Jangira, N. K. (1987). Education for Rehabilitation of the Disabled.*Indian Journal of Disability and Rehabilitation*, 1, 9-12.

Jangira, N. K., and Mani, M. N. G. (1990). *Integrated Education for Visually Handicapped: Management Perspective*. Delhi: Academic Press.

Jangira, N.K., 'Special Educational Needs of Children and Young Adults: An Unfinished Agenda,' *Education and Children with Special Needs: From Segregation to Inclusion*, Ed. Seamus Hegarty, Mithu Alur, Thousand Oaks: Sage Publications Inc., 1997. Print.

Janshala (2003). *Perspectives in special needs education in India. A journey from isolation to inclusion.* Jan.-March.

Johnson, W. D., and Johnson, T. R. (1990). Integrating Handicapped Students into the mainstream.*Exceptional Children*, 47, 2, 90-99.

Kalyanpur, Maya. 'Equality, Quality and Quantity: Challenges in Inclusive Education Policy and Service Provision in India.' *International Journal of Inclusive Education*. 12.3 (2008): Print.

Kapperman, G, Sticken, J, and Heinze, T. (2002). Survey of the use of assistive technology by Illinois students who are visually impaired. *Journal of Visual Impairment and Blindness*, 96, 106-108.

Karna, G.N. (1999). *United Nations and Rights of Disabled Persons: A Study in Indian Perspective*. New Delhi: A.P.H. Publishing Corporation.

Karna, G.N. (2001). *Disability Studies in India: Retrospect and Prospects*. New Delhi: Gyan Publishing House.

Kauffman, J.M. and Hallahan, D. P. (1981). *Handbook of Special Education*. New Delhi: Prentice-Hall.

Kauffman, M.J., Gottlieb, J., Agard, J. A., and Kukic, M. B. (1975). Mainstreaming: Toward an explication of the construct. *Focus on Exceptional Children*, 7, 1-12.

Kelly, S. M. and Smith, D.W. (2011). The impact of assistive technology on the educational performance of students with visual impairments: A synthesis of the research. *Journal of Visual Impairment and Blindness*, 105, 73-83.

Kelly, S.M. (2008). Correlates of assistive technology use by students who are visually impaired in the U.S.: Multilevel modeling of the Special Education Elementary Longitudinal Study. Unpublished dissertation.Northern Illinois University, Illinois.

Kirk, S. A., and Gallagher. (1979). *Educating Exceptional Children*. Boston: Houghton Mifflin Co.

Kundu, C. L. (2000). *Status of Disability in India 2000*. New Delhi: Rehabilitation Council of India.

Leicester, M. (1999). Disability Voice: Towards an enabling education. In T. Cook, J. Swain and S. French, Voices from Segregated Schooling: towards an inclusive education system. *Disability and Society*, 16, 2, 293-310.

Llewwllyn, A., and Hogan, K. (200). The Use and Abuse of Models of Disability. *Disability and Society*, 15, 1, 157-165.

Lowenfeld, B. (1973). *The Visually Handicapped Child in School*. New York: John Day.

Mani, D. R. (1988). *The Physically Handicapped in India: Policy and Programme*. New Delhi: Ashish Publications.

Mead, G.H. (1934). *Mind, Self and Society*. Chicago: University of Chicago Press.

Miles, M. (1995). Disability in an Eastern Religious Context: historical perspectives. Ministry of Human Resource Development (2004). *Education for all: India Marches Ahead*. New Delhi: Government of India.

Murphy, J., Hatton, D., and Erickson, K.A. (2008). Exploring early literacy practices of teachers of infants, toddlers, and preschoolers with visual impairments. *Journal of Visual Impairment and Blindness*, 102, 133-146.

Oliver, M. (1983). *Social Work with Disabled People*. London: The MacMillan Press Ltd.

Oliver, M. (1990). *The Politics of Disablement*. London: MacMillan Press.

Oliver, M. (1995). *Understanding Disability: From Theory to Practice* Basingstoke : MacMillan.

Oliver, M., and Zarb, G. (1989). The Politics of Disability: A New Approach. *Disability, Handicap and Society*, 4, 3, 221-239.

Pal, G. (2000). Education of the Disabled: The Shifting Paradigms. *Perspectives in Education*, 18, 1, 31-42.

Parker, S., Buckley, W., Truesdell, A., Riggio, M., Collins, M., and Boardman, B. (1990). Barriers to the use of assistive technology with children: A Survey. *Journal of Visual Impairment and Blindness*, 84, 532-533.

Parson, T. (1951). *The Social System*. London: Routledge.

Paterson, K. and Hughes, B. (1999). Disability studies and phenomenology: the carnal politics of everyday life, *Disability and Society*, 14, 5, 597–611.

Pijl, S. J., and Meyer, C.J.W. (1991). Does Integration count for much? An analysis of the practice of integration in eight countries.*European Journal of Special Needs Education*, 6, 2, 100-110.

Pijl, S. J., Meyer, C.J.W., and Hegarty, S. (1997). *A Global Agenda*. London: Routledge.

Priestley, M. (1998). Constructions and Creations: idealism, materialism and disability theory. *Disability and Society*, 13, 1, 75-94.

Quinn, G. (1995). The International Convention on Civil and Political Rights and disability: a conceptual framework. In G. N. Karna, *United Nations and Rights of Disabled Persons: A Study in Indian Perspective*. New Delhi: A.P.H. Publishing Corporation.

Quinn, P. (1998). *Understanding Disability: A Life Approach*. New Delhi: Sage.

Reindal, S.M. (1995). Discussing Disability: An investigation into theories of Disability.*European Journal of Special Needs Education*, 10, 1, 58-69.

Reynolds, M.C., and Wang, M.C. (1983). Restructuring 'special' education school programs: A position paper. *Policy Studies Review*, 2, 1, 189-212.

Reynolds, M.C., Wang, M.C., and Walberg, H.J. (1987). The Necessary Restructuring of Special and Regular Education. *Exceptional Children*, 53, 5, 391-398.

Rhodes, D. (1985). *An Outline of History Medicine*. London: Butterworth.

Safilos-Rothschild, C. (1970) *The Sociology and Social Psychology of Disability and Rehabilitation*. New York: Random House.

Sahfi, M. Y, Zhou, L, Smith, D. W, and Kelley, P. (2009). Assistive technology in teacher-training programmes: A national and international perspective. *Journal of Visual Impairment and Blindness*, 103, 562-568.

Seetharam, M. (1982). *Study of the Centrally Sponsored Scheme of Integrated Education for Handicapped Children in Normal Schools in Delhi*. New Delhi: Council for Social Development.

Shakespeare, T. (1994). Cultural Representation of disabled People: dustbins or disapproval? *Disability and Society*, 9, 3, 283-301.

Shakespeare, T. (1997, December).'Researching Disabled Sexuality'. In C. Barnes, *A Working Social Model? Disability and Work in the 21st Century*. Paper presented at the Disability Studies Conference and Seminar, Edinburgh.

Smith, D.W, Kelley, P., Maushak, N. J., Griffin-Shirley, N., and Lan, W. Y. (2009). Assistive technology competencies for teachers of students with visual impairments. *Journal of Visual Impairment and Blindness*, 103, 457-469.

Soder, M. (1989). Disability as a social construct: the labelling approach revisited. *European Journal of Special Needs Education*, 4, 2, 117-129.

Soder, M. (1991). Theory, ideology and research: A response to Tony Booth. *European Journal of Special Needs Education*, 6, 1, 17-23.

Stangvik, G. (1997). Beyond Schooling: Integration in a Policy Perspective. In S, Pijl., C.J.W. Meyer., and S. Hegarty, S. *A Global Agenda*. London: Routledge.

Swain, J., Finkelstein, V., French, S. and Oliver, M. (1993). *Disabling Barriers-Enabling Environments*. London: Sage

The Salamanca Statement and Framework for Action on Special Needs Education; Adopted by World Conference in Special Needs Education: Access and Quality. Salamanca, Spain; 7-10 June 1994.

Tomlinson, S. (1982). *A Sociology of Special Education*. London: Routledge and Kegan Paul.

Tregaskis, C. (2002). Social Model Theory: The story so far... *Disability and Society*, 17, 4, 457-470.

Tuttle, D.W. (1987). The Role of the Special Educators, Teacher-Counsellor in Meeting Students' Self Esteem Needs. *Journal of Visual Impairment and Blindness*, 81, 4, 156-161.

UN Convention for Protection of Rights of Disabled Persons. Convention and Optional Protocol Signatures and Ratifications, 30.3.2007.

UN Convention for Protection of Rights of Disabled Persons. Convention and Optional Protocol Signatures and Ratifications, 1.10.2007.

UNESCO (1999). *Salamanca Five Years On: A Review of UNESCO Activities in the Light of the Salamanca Statement Framework of Action of Special Needs Education.* Paris: UNESCO.

UPIAS. (1976). 'Fundamental Principles of Disability'. London: Union of the Physically Impaired Against Segregation.

Wilson, D. H. (2012). High-tech implants will soon be commonplace enhancements under our skin and inside our skulls, making us stronger and smarter. Daniel H. Wilson on our 'superabled' future.The Wall Street Journal, June 1.

World Bank (2007): *People with Disabilities in India: From Commitments to Outcomes*, Human Development Unit, South Asia Region, The World Bank, New Delhi.

World Health Organisation. (1980). *The International Classification of Impairments, Disabilities and Handicaps*. Geneva: WHO.

World Health Organisation.(2001). *International Classification of Functioning, Disability and Health*. Geneva: WHO.

Appendices

Appendix A

Developmental Milestones for Infants with Visual Impairments

Developmental Area	Birth-12 months	13-24 months	25-36 months
Cognitive	* Imitates sounds, gestures, or actions * Shows displeasure at loss of toy or object * Demonstrates object permanence * Begins to demonstrate cause and effect or means-end behaviors	* Imitates use of toy * Points to body parts * Demonstrates (e.g., sings a song) * Uses objects as tools * Uses trial and error	* Matches objects * Remembers past events * Begins to sort objects by size, color, texture and shape * Tells use of objects
Communication	* Smiles * Makes eye or face contact * Babbles * Laughs * Says first word * Understands "no" * Responds	* Uses gestures (points, waves) * Uses 2-word sentences * Follows sim ple directions * Names familiar objects and people	* Uses first person pronouns (I, me) * Asks questions * Understands some prepositions (on, next to, on top of) * Begins to use imagination
Gross Motor (large muscles)	* Controls head (holds upright when being held or when lying on tummy) * Rolls over * Sits * Crawls	* Pulls to stand * Walks * Climbs into adult-size chairs * Rolls, then throws ball	* Walks up and down stairs * Begins to run * Begins to jump * Balances on one foot
Fine Motor (small muscles)	* Brings hands together * Grasps objects * Reaches for toys (either visually or auditorally) * Searches for a dropped toy * Explores objects (pats, pokes, hits together)	* Releases objects on purpose * Uses pincer grasp (thumb and index finger) * Scribbles * Puts objects inside containers * Completes simple form board puzzles * Turns pages of books * Uses wrist rotation (turns doorknobs, jar lids, etc.)	* Stacks objects * Copies geometric figures (either tactually or visually) * Strings beads * Sorts objects by size and texture

Developmental Area	Birth-12 months	13-24 months	25-36 months
Self-Help	* Eats with spoon * Holds and drinks from bottle * Eats some finger foods	* Drinks from cup * Removes some clothing independently * Indicates toilet needs * Anticipates some daily routines	* Puts on some clothing independently * Puts toys away * Partially or fully toilet trained
Sensory	* Focuses on and follows objects * Turns to sound * Explores objects by touch	* Identifies hot and cold * Identifies familiar sounds * Identifies familiar odours * Recognizes objects by touch * Explores objects or surfaces with feet	* Recognizes places or activities by odors or sounds * "Tracks" Braille (follows along in book or on label) * Identifies textures
Social	* Makes eye or face contact * Smiles * Recognizes parents and family members * Reaches for familiar person * Cries when parent leaves	* Plays interactive games with adults * Hugs * Repeats actions that others laugh at * Imitates household activities (feeding baby, sweeping, etc.)-fantasy play * Plays independently	* Plays interactively with peers * Shows signs of ownership * Asks for help * Pretends

Appendix B

Checklist for the Teachers for Observation of Symptoms that may Indicate a Visual Problem

- Frequent sites.
- Tendency to rub at eyes.
- Tilting or nodding head when looking at objects.
- Squinting, blinking, twitching of eyes.
- Extreme sensitivity to light.
- Inflamed, running eyes; red-rimmed or swollen lids.
- Crossed eyes.
- Eyeballs smaller or larger than usual.
- Sunken eyeballs.
- Unusual eye movements.
- Lack of sustained fixation on target or lack of eye contact.
- Student avoids close work.
- Student displays tension during close work.
- Delayed response when visual materials are presented.
- Tendency to close one eye when looking at materials.

- Appears to look left or right of objects instead of looking directly at them.
- Holds the page too close or too far away when reading (normal distance is about 16 inches from the eyes).
- Excessive head movements while reading.
- Complaint of blurring when viewing materials near or far.
- Complaint of headaches, dizziness or nausea associated with the use of the eyes.
- Complaint of pain or discomfort in eyes.
- Complaint of seeing double.
- Complaint of not being able to see straight ahead, on the sides or in one visual area.
- Excessive reversals in reading.
- Loses place while reading.
- Skips lines unknowingly.
- Does not follow lines in exercise books.
- Complaint of words or letters running together.
- Thrusting head forward when observing distant objects.
- Impaired colour perception.
- Poor eye and hand coordination.
- Uneven gait and/or difficulty in moving around the room or school.
- Frequent stumbling when moving.
- Has difficulty seeing or moving at night or in darkened areas.
- Has difficulty moving from bright to dark or dim areas.

Appendix C

Eye Conditions

Achromatopsia (uh-krome-uh-**tope**-see-uh)

Rod Monochromatism (mon-o-**krome**-uh-tiz-um)

What is achromatopsia?

Achromatopsia (also known as rod monochromatism) is a rare genetic eye disorder which is present from birth and results in little or no function of the cone cells of the retina (back wall of the eye). In the normal eye, there are about six million cone receptors located mostly at the centre of the retina. Cones permit light adaptation, colour perception and perception of fine detail. Individuals with achromatopsia are either partially or totally colour blind. Their eyes cannot adapt normally to lighting brighter than twilight conditions. Since cones are located in the area of the retina responsible for central vision, the result is reduced visual acuity which cannot be corrected by glasses or contact lenses.

What are the characteristics of achromatopsia?

- Possiblenystagmus (uncontrolled movement of the eyes).
- Possible difficulty or inability to see colors.
- Extreme photophobia (sensitivity to light).
- Near vision is generally less affected than distance vision.

- Student will see best in the evening or in dimly lit environments.
- Visual acuity is reduced and not able to be corrected with glasses or contact lenses.

What are the functional implications of achromatopsia?

- Student will experience fluctuating visual functioning depending on lighting.
- Student may not be able to move safely through his or her environment.
- Visual tasks will cause fatigue.
- Glare must be avoided.
- Rest periods may be needed when doing close work.
- Low vision aids may be needed.

What are some educational considerations for a student with achromatopsia?

- Print materials may need to be enlarged with high contrast.
- Dark-lined exercise books and black felt tip pens may be beneficial.
- Lighting will be a major factor in the student's visual functioning.
- Care must be taken that tasks requiring colour vision are adapted/modified.
- Student may need extra time to complete visual tasks.
- Student may benefit from breaks from visual tasks to combat eye fatigue.
- Student may require orientation and mobility training.
- Physical activities may need to be restricted for safety.
- Student may need to sit closer to chalkboard and demonstrations.
- Low vision aids may be helpful.
- Student may need time to adjust to changes in lighting.
- Student must be permitted to wear sunglasses, visors, etc. In school, if desired.

- Student must be asked for his or her own preferences regarding lighting, seating, magnification, etc..

Aniridia (an-er-id-ee-uh)

What is aniridia?

Aniridia is a rare, hereditary condition in which the iris does not completely form. The iris is the coloured part of the eye. It controls the amount of light entering the eye by varying the degree of the pupillary opening. Aniridia is often accompanied by cataract formation and/or glaucoma.

What are the characteristics of aniridia?

- Decreased visual acuity.
- Nystagmus.
- Photophobia (extreme sensitivity to light).
- Field loss corresponding to the area where the iris is absent.
- Cataracts and glaucoma frequently present.
- Fluctuating vision depending on lighting conditions and glare.

What are the functional implications of aniridia?

- Orientation and mobility will be of concern.
- Glare must be avoided.
- Use of low vision aids may be helpful.
- Lighting will be a major factor in visual functioning.
- Student will need time to adapt to changes in lighting; recovery from glare is slow.
- Eye fatigue may be a concern.

What are some educational considerations for a student with aniridia?

- Student will need lighting considerations (normal or dim lighting may be preferable).
- Student may need extra time to complete visual tasks.
- Large print and high contrast materials may be helpful.

- Student may need to sit closer to the board or demonstrations.
- Student may need to use black felt pen or marker for writing.
- Student may need to use dark-lined paper.
- Training in the area of orientation and mobility will be necessary.
- Student may benefit from breaks from visual tasks to combat eye fatigue.
- Stress will complicate nystagmus, therefore assignments and writing tasks should be asbrief as possible.
- Keyboarding skills will likely be important as students may have difficulty with handwriting.
- Use of low vision aids may be helpful.
- Glare should be avoided in all situations.
- Student may benefit from a tilted reading stand.
- Student may need to use sunglasses or visors for light sensitivity.
- Student may need time to allow eyes to adjust to changes in lighting.

Cataracts (kat-er-acts)

What are cataracts?

Cataracts are opacities (cloudiness, fogginess) of the lens which restrict the passage of light into the eye, thus preventing a clear image from forming on the retina (back wall of the eye). Cataracts may be congenital or adventitious, progressive or nonprogressive. They may becaused by injury or trauma, some eye diseases (glaucoma, retinitis pigmentosa, etc.), intrauterine infections, aging or heredity. Visual fields are usually normal, and severe cases may be accompanied by nystagmus (uncontrolled movement of the eyes). Cataracts may be surgically removed, and wearing eye glasses or contact lenses will compensate for the loss of the lens. Artificial lenses may also be implanted in some children. Aphakia (uh-fake-ee-uh) refers to the condition in which the lens has been surgically removed from the eye.

What are the characteristics of cataracts?

- Student may exhibit nystagmus.
- Student may experience blurred vision.
- A milky white spot may be visible in the student's pupil.
- Student may exhibit photophobia (extreme sensitivity to light) and/or distorted colorvision.
- If cataracts are not surgically corrected, amblyopia (lazy eye') may develop.
- Student may experience double vision.

What are the functional implications of cataracts?

- Student may utilise eccentric viewing (turning head or body to see).
- Student may not be able to move safely through his or her environment.
- Visual tasks will cause fatigue.
- Glare must be avoided.
- Rest periods may be needed when doing close work.
- Visual functioning may fluctuate depending on maturity of cataracts.
- If wearing strong eyeglasses ('coke bottle' lenses), the student may have restricted peripheral vision.

What are some educational considerations for a student with cataracts?

- High contrast materials will be beneficial.
- Lighting will be a major factor in the student's visual functioning.
- Student may need extra time to complete visual tasks.
- Student may benefit from breaks from visual tasks to combat eye fatigue.
- Student may require orientation and mobility training.
- Physical activities may need to be restricted for safety.
- Print materials may need to be enlarged and high contrast

materials provided.

- Dark-lined exercise books and black felt-tip pens may be helpful.
- Low vision aids may be useful.
- Student may need time to adjust to changes in lighting.
- Student may need to sit closer to chalkboard or demonstrations.
- Student may benefit from wearing specially colored (noir orange) lenses.
- Teacher should not stand in front of the window or other light source.

Astigmatism (uh-stig-muh-ti-zum)

What is astigmatism?

Astigmatism is an irregular curvature of the cornea (or lens) of the eye. The primary cause ofastigmatism is the cornea being shaped more like a football than being rounded. Light entering the eye will not be bent equally in all directions, resulting in distorted vision. Regular stigmatism may be simple or compound and frequently accompanies myopia (near-sightedness) and yperopia (far-sightedness). Regular types may often be remediated using corrective lenses. Irregular astigmatism would result when the cornea has been damaged by trauma, inflammation, scar tissueor developmental problems. This type may not always be corrected completely by correctivelenses.

What are the characteristics of astigmatism?

- Clear visual acuity may not be possible.
- Depth perception may be affected.
- Physical activities may be restricted.
- Corrective lenses may be necessary to achieve optimum vision.

What are the functional implications of astigmatism?

- Glare must be avoided.

- High contrast materials are important.
- Orientation and mobility skills may be of concern.
- Use of certain low vision aids may be helpful.
- Lighting will be a major factor in visual functioning.
- Lack of depth perception may cause some difficulty.
- Student may have sensitivity to certain levels or types of light.
- Visual fatigue may be experienced when performing visual tasks.
- Doing close work and reading may cause headaches.

What are some educational considerations for a student with astigmatism?

- Student will need lighting considerations.
- Student may need extra time to complete visual tasks.
- Student may need to sit closer to the board or demonstrations.
- Student may need assistance or alternate ways to take notes.
- Student may need to use black felt pen, marker and/or dark-lined paper for writing.
- Student may benefit from breaks from visual tasks to combat eye fatigue.
- Student may require orientation and mobility training.
- Physical activities may need to be restricted.
- Using colour computer monitors may be useful for some students.
- A slanted or tilted reading stand may be helpful.

Amblyopia (am-blee-ope-ee-uh)

What is amblyopia?

Amblyopia, or 'lazy eye,' is a condition in which one of the eyes has poor vision although there is no disease or malformation of that eye. If the eyes are not straight (strabismus), the student may suppress the vision in the turning eye to avoid seeing double. In other cases, the two eyes may be seeing quite differently due to the presence of unequal refractive errors (near-sightedness or far-sightedness). In all cases of amblyopia, the brain 'shuts off' one eye to favour the eye with better vision. Amblyopia may be treated by patching the good eye, by surgery or with corrective lenses.

What are the characteristics of amblyopia?

- Eyes may not be straight.
- Depth perception may be reduced or absent.
- Disturbance in vision.
- Visual acuity is likely less than average, particularly in near vision.

What are the functional implications of amblyopia?

- Depth perception may be reduced or absent.
- Student may have difficulty discerning fine details.
- Student may have difficulty with fine motor skills.
- Student may require wearing a patch, which would result in decreased vision initially.
- Student may have self-esteem issues because he or she looks different.
- Student may possibly have field loss.

What are some educational considerations for a student with amblyopia?

- Large print and high contrast materials may be helpful.
- Student may need to sit closer to the board or demonstrations.
- Student may have difficulty with fine motor skills such as cutting paper, coloring or printing within lines.
- Student may need to use black felt pen or marker for writing.
- Reading/writing sessions should be kept as brief as possible when student is wearing apatch to reduce eye fatigue.

- Tasks requiring depth perception, such as catching a ball or moving in uneven terrain, may be difficult.
- Classmates may benefit from an explanation about the patch so that the student is made to feel comfortable.
- Mobility around school and playground may need to be monitored due to reduced depth perception.
- Preferential lighting may be considered.
- Glare should be avoided.
- Student may need familiarisation with the environment to help anticipate distances and heights.

Cortical Visual Impairment (CVI)

What is cortical visual impairment?

Cortical visual impairment (CVI) is a condition in which the vision is reduced, but the vision loss can not be explained by ophthalmological findings. The eyes appear normal and capable of functioning, but the brain does not process the visual information which it is given. There is usually clinical evidence of damage to the cortical area of the brain (the outer layer of gray matter over most of the brain). The process of receiving visual information may be disturbed, the interpretation of that information may be disturbed or there may be a combination of both. CVI may be caused by a great variety of diseases and disorders such as malformation of the brain, lack of oxygen at birth or later in life, head injury and infections such as meningitis. Children with CVI will usually have additional neurological difficulties such as cerebral palsy, seizures or developmental delay. There are, however, children with CVI who have no additional disabilities. Children with CVI usually have residual vision, but their visual functioning is extremely variable and fluctuates. Visual functioning may improve in some children as further cognitive development occurs.

What are the characteristics of cortical visual impairment?

- Student will have extremely variable visual functioning (day to day, hour to hour).

- Student will exhibit visual inattention or lack of visual curiosity.
- Students will usually see better in familiar environments and with familiar objects.
- Student will not 'look blind'—eyes appear normal and appear to be focussed.
- Student will not often exhibit self stimulating behaviours.
- Student will seem to recognise (primary) colours more easily than shapes.
- Student may see moving objects more easily than stationary objects.
- Student may look to the side when reaching in order to use peripheral vision.
- Student may have difficulty crossing mid-line.

What are the functional implications of cortical visual impairment?

- Student will need flexibility in his or her programming to accommodate fluctuating vision.
- Student may not move safely through his or her environment.
- Visual clutter must be avoided to minimise distraction.
- Care must be taken to avoid overloading the student with visual information.
- Student will need to make maximum use of all his or her senses.
- Student will benefit from consistent repetition of tasks and routines.

What are some educational considerations for a student with cortical visual impairment?

- High contrast materials will be beneficial.
- Use primary colours to outline simple shapes to make them more visible.
- Student may need extra time to complete visual tasks.

- Give student time to process visual information.
- Use familiar objects in familiar environments.
- Keep the number of people working with the student to a minimum.
- Keep visual information simple, constant and predictable.
- Student may benefit from breaks from visual tasks to combat eye fatigue.
- Encourage student to explore what he or she sees.
- Lighting will be a factor in the student's visual functioning.
- Student may require orientation and mobility training.

Hemianopsia (he-mee-in-op-see-uh)

What is hemianopsia?

Hemianopsia is a condition in which there is blindness or impaired vision in one half of thevisual field (literally, 'half vision'). Hemianopsia may be caused by factors such as stroke, tumor or traumatic brain injury affecting the optic nerve. The particular portion of the visual field affected depends on the site of the damage. One or both eyes may be affected, and acuity usually is not affected in the intact portion of the visual field.

What are the characteristics of hemianopsia?

- Student may frequently bump into objects.
- Student may exhibit possible blurring in specific areas of his or her vision.
- Depending on site of lesson, student may have difficulty with speech and language, ability to concentrate, and visual attention.
- Student may seem hesitant to move with ease through his or her environment.
- Night vision may be reduced.

What are the functional implications of hemianopsia?

- Visual fatigue may be experienced when performing visual tasks.

- Reading speed is reduced and strategies need to be taught to help the student find information on the page.
- Reading ability may be affected to such a degree that audio taped materials may be useful.
- Student may use eccentric viewing (turning the head or body to facilitate seeing).
- Student may not move efficiently or safely through environment.
- Scanning and tracking is difficult.

What are some educational considerations for a student with hemianopsia?

- Student may benefit from using mirrors and/or prisms.
- Visual clutter should be avoided.
- Student may need extra time to complete visual tasks.
- Student may need assistance or alternate ways to take notes.
- Student may benefit from breaks from visual tasks to combat eye fatigue.
- Student may require orientation and mobility training.
- Skills needed for reading may need to be specifically taught (e.g., scanning, tracking, keeping place on page, finding information on page, etc.).
- Care should be taken to accommodate the student's attention span, frustration level andother such characteristics when assigning tasks.
- Student may benefit from training in techniques of eccentric viewing (turning the head orbody to facilitate better viewing).

Glaucoma (glah-ko-muh)

What is glaucoma?

Glaucoma is a disease in which increased pressure of the fluid inside the eye (intraocular pressure) causes degeneration of the optic disk and visual field loss. The fluid inside the eye is called the aqueous humour. It carries nutrients to the front part of the eye and is then drained into the blood stream through a channel called the canal of Schlemm. In glaucoma, the canal of Schlemm becomes blocked, causing a buildup of pressure within the eye. When intraocular pressure is too high, it is difficult for the blood to supply the retina and optic nerve nutritionally. This results in a reduction in the visual field and in visual acuity. There are four types of glaucoma: chronic open angle, acute angle closure, congenital and secondary. Glaucoma may be treated with medications or surgery. Vision loss due to glaucoma is not reversible.

What are the characteristics of glaucoma?

- If chronic open angle glaucoma, the student may not exhibit physical symptoms untilvisual impairment occurs.
- If acute angle closure glaucoma, the student may experience sudden onset of blurred vision followed by excruciating pain, nausea and vomiting, redness of the eye, cloudy vision and a multi-coloured halo may be seen around lights.
- If congenital glaucoma, the child may present as photophobic (extremely sensitive tolight) and may have excessive tearing and cloudiness of the cornea.
- If secondary glaucoma, student will have had an eye insult or injury, or will be reacting to another disorder such as cataract surgery, infection, aniridia, medication, etc..
- Student may describe blurring in specific areas of their vision.
- Depending on site of lesson, student may have difficulty with speech and language, ability to concentrate and visual attention.
- Student may not move with ease through his or her environment.
- Night vision may be reduced.

What are the functional implications of glaucoma?

- Student may have poor night vision and poor peripheral fields.

- Student may exhibit photophobia (extreme sensitivity to light).
- Reading or seeing large objects at close range may be difficult.
- Medications needed to treat glaucoma may require monitoring.
- Visual functioning may fluctuate.
- Student may present with headaches, pain, redness of the eye, cloudy cornea and/or wide open pupil.

What are some educational considerations for a student with glaucoma?

- Student may need extra time to complete visual tasks.
- Student may need assistance or alternate ways to take notes.
- Student may benefit from breaks from visual tasks to combat eye fatigue.
- Print materials which are enlarged and high contrast will be necessary.
- Lighting will be a major factor in the student's visual functioning.
- Glare should be avoided and bright lights may not be tolerated.
- Use of low vision aids may be beneficial for some students.
- Use of closed circuit television (cctv) may be beneficial.
- Student may require orientation and mobility training for night travelling.
- Physical activities may need to be restricted; check with the student's ophthalmologist.

Leber's (lay-bers) Optic Atrophy

What is Leber's Optic Atrophy?

Leber's Optic Atrophy is a condition in which there is rapidly progressive optic atrophy (degeneration of nerve tissue which carries optic messages to the brain). This is a rare disease which occurs mostly in young men aged 20-30 years and is hereditary (due to an X-linked recessive gene). The disease may include other types of central nervous system involvement.

What are the characteristics of Leber's Optic Atrophy?

- Decreased visual acuity in central field.
- Fluctuating visual performance.
- Colour vision may be reduced.
- Visual perception may be impaired.
- Eye fatigue when performing visual tasks.

What are the functional implications of Leber's Optic Atrophy?

- Orientation and mobility will likely be of concern.
- Depth perception may be affected.
- Glare must be avoided.
- Use of low vision aids may be helpful in some situations.
- Lighting will be a major factor in visual functioning.
- Student may have sensitivity to certain levels or types of light.

What are some educational considerations for a student with Leber's Optic Atrophy?

- Student will need lighting considerations.
- Student may need extra time to complete visual tasks.
- Large print, high contrast and audiotaped materials may be helpful.
- Student may need to learn braille.
- Student may need to sit closer to the board or demonstrations.
- Student may need to use black felt pen or marker for writing.
- Student may need to use dark-lined paper.
- Avoid visual clutter.
- Student may benefit from breaks from visual tasks to combat eye fatigue.

- Glare should be avoided in all situations.
- Teacher needs to be aware that student's visual functioning may fluctuate, therefore, so should expectations.
- Student may benefit from use of low vision aids.
- Student will require orientation and mobility training.
- Keyboarding skills may be necessary.
- Student may need time to adjust to changes in lighting.
- Physical activity may be restricted; check with the student's ophthalmologist.

Hyperopia (hipe-er-ope-ee-uh)

What is hyperopia?

Hyperopia, commonly referred to as 'farsightedness,' is an eye condition in which light rays from distant objects do not converge soon enough to focuss on the retina. It causes the individual to not be able to see things close to them as clearly as things which are farther away from them. It is a refractive error and is related to shortness of the eyeball or to reduced curvatures of the cornea or lens. Hyperopia may be progressive or not and may affect individuals of any age. Convex or 'plus' lenses correct this difficulty.

What are the characteristics of hyperopia?

- Clear visual acuity may not be possible.
- Student may bring objects in close to his or her face in order to focus, thus appearing to be very near-sighted.
- Corrective lenses are necessary to achieve optimum vision.
- Student may squint or frown in an attempt to narrow. what he or she sees because it is easier to see that way.

What are the functional implications of hyperopia?

- High contrast materials are important.
- Use of certain low vision aids may be helpful.
- Lighting will be a major factor in visual functioning.
- Visual fatigue may be experienced when performing near vision tasks.

- Student may complain of eye-strain.
- Performing visual tasks may cause headaches.
- Student may avoid near vision tasks such as reading.

What are some educational considerations for a student with hyperopia?

- Glare must be avoided.
- Student will need lighting considerations.
- Care must be taken to provide student with high contrast print materials.
- Student may need extra time to complete visual tasks.
- Student may need to sit further away from the board or demonstrations.
- Student may need assistance or alternate ways to take notes.
- Student may need to use black felt pen, marker and/or dark-lined paper for writing.
- Student may benefit from breaks from visual tasks to combat eye fatigue.
- Student may require orientation and mobility training.
- Physical activities may be preferred to visual activities.
- Where possible, student should be given opportunities for manipulation of concrete objects instead of pencil and paper tasks.

Myopia (my-ope-ee-uh)

What is myopia?

Myopia, commonly referred to as 'near-sightedness' or 'short-sightedness,' is an eye condition in which light rays from distant objects converge too soon to focuss on the retina. It causes the individual to not be able to see things far away from them as clearly as things which are close to them. It is a refractive error and is related to extra length of the eyeball or to increased curvatures of the cornea or lens. Myopia may be progressive or not and may affect individuals of any age. Concave or 'minus' lenses correct this difficulty. Individuals with high myopia may be at increased risk for retinal detachment.

What are the characteristics of myopia?

- Clear visual acuity may not be possible.
- Student may bring objects in close to his or her face in order to focuss.
- Corrective lenses are necessary to achieve optimum vision.
- Student may not be interested in activities which require distance vision, particularly physical education activities.
- Night vision may be poor.

What are the functional implications of myopia?

- High contrast materials are important.
- Use of certain low vision aids may be helpful.
- Lighting will be a major factor in visual functioning.
- Visual fatigue may be experienced when performing visual tasks.
- Student may complain of eye-strain.
- Performing visual tasks may cause headaches

What are some educational considerations for a student with myopia?

- Glare must be avoided.
- Student will need lighting considerations.
- Care must be taken to provide student with high contrast print materials.
- Student may need extra time to complete visual tasks.
- Student may need to sit closer to the board or demonstrations.
- Student may need assistance or alternate ways to take notes.
- Student may need to use black felt pen, marker and/or dark-line paper for writing.

- Student may benefit from breaks from visual tasks to combat eye fatigue.
- Student may require orientation and mobility training.
- Physical activities may need to be restricted; check with the student's ophthalmologist.
- Where possible, student should be given opportunities for manipulation of concrete objects instead of pencil and paper tasks.

Macular (mak-you-ler) Degeneration

What is macular degeneration?

Macular degeneration is a condition in which there is progressive degenerative damage to the central part of the retina, the macula. There are two types: juvenile (less than seven years of age) or senile. The latter is commonly present in elders, but sometimes is present in children. Associated with macular degeneration is central field loss, which affects acuity and colour vision. Peripheral vision is normal. The condition also causes light sensitivity.

What are the characteristics of macular degeneration?

- Decreased visual acuity in central field.
- Loss of central vision while peripheral vision is normal.
- Colour vision reduced.
- Photophobia (extreme sensitivity to light).
- May need to use eccentric viewing (tilting or turning head to find best viewing position).
- Eye fatigue when performing visual tasks.

What are the functional implications of macular degeneration?

- Orientation and mobility will be of concern.
- Training in daily living skills may be necessary.
- Glare must be avoided.
- Use of low vision aids may be helpful in some situations.
- Lighting will be a major factor in visual functioning.

- Student may have self-esteem issues due to use of eccentric viewing.

What are some educational considerations for a students with macular degeneration?

- Student will need average or dim lighting.
- Student may need extra time to complete tasks.
- Large print, high contrast and audio-taped materials may be helpful.
- Student may need to use black felt pen or marker for writing.
- Student may need to sit near board or demonstrations.
- Training in the area of orientation and mobility will be necessary.
- Use of low vision aids may be helpful.
- Glare should be avoided in all situations.
- Student may benefit from a tilted reading stand.
- Student may need to use sun-glasses or visors for light sensitivity.
- Student may need to learn organised search patterns to locate objects or visual targets.
- Materials which require colour vision should be adapted or not used.
- Student may use eccentric viewing and classmates should know why.
- Training may be necessary in daily living skills.
- Student may benefit from adjustment to blindness counselling.

Coloboma (ko-luh-bo-muh)

What is coloboma?

Coloboma is a rare, congenital condition in which there is a cleft or defect in a part of the eye. It sometimes involves the iris, retina, optic nerve or optic disk. A coloboma is sometimes accompanied by glaucoma or cataracts. A coloboma may have minor or major effect on visual functioning.

What are the characteristics of coloboma?

- Decreased visual acuity which varies according to the number of parts of the eye affected.
- Possible peripheral or central field loss if coloboma extends to the retina.
- Possible nystagmus.
- Photophobia (extreme sensitivity to light).
- Cataracts and glaucoma may be present.
- Possible problems with depth perception.
- Eye fatigue likely.

What are the functional implications of coloboma?

- Glare must be avoided.
- Use of low vision aids may be helpful.
- Lighting will be a major factor in visual functioning.
- Eye fatigue may be a concern.
- Depth perception may be affected.

What are some educational considerations for a student with coloboma?

- Student will need lighting considerations.
- Student may need extra time to complete visual tasks.
- Large print and high contrast materials may be helpful.
- Student may need to sit closer to the board or demonstrations.
- Student may need to use black felt pen or marker for writing.
- Student may need to use dark-lined paper.
- Student may benefit from breaks from visual tasks to combat eye fatigue.
- Glare should be avoided in all situations.

- Student may benefit from a tilted reading stand.
- Student may need to use sun-glasses or visors for light sensitivity.
- Student may benefit from orientation and mobility training because of depth perception and field loss.
- Keyboarding skills may be helpful if student experiences difficulty with handwriting.

Nystagmus (ni-stag-mus)

What is nystagmus?

Nystagmus means the rhythmical, involuntary movement of one or both eyes. It is a physical sign of utmost importance because it can signal the presence of other eye conditions. It can be so slight that it is hardly noticeable or it can be rapid with a wide range of movement. It is really a defence mechanism of the muscles of the eyes in search of fixation (focuss) and orientation in space.

What are the characteristics of nystagmus?

- Involuntary, rhythmic movement of the eyes which can be horizontal, vertical, rotary or mixed.
- Two types: Congenital (most common in children) and acquired (not present at birth).
- Most frequently occurs in both eyes and is usually a connected movement.
- Possible head tilting and nodding.
- Possible dizziness.
- Possible disturbance in vision.
- Clarity is always less than average, particularly in near vision.
- May be more noticeable when the student is sick or tired.

What are some functional implications of nystagmus?

- Student often experiences myopia ('near-sightedness') resulting in reduced visual acuity.

- Student experiences eye fatigue when asked to use vision continuously.
- Student may experience vertigo.
- Stress or spinning movements increase nystagmus and should be avoided when fixation is required.
- Head tilting may decrease nystagmus and is usually involuntary.
- Student may exhibit head nodding.

What are some educational considerations for a student with nystagmus?

- Large print materials may be helpful.
- Magnifiers may not always be helpful.
- Print materials should be as uncluttered as possible.
- Line markers, line guides or rulers may help student keep place on the page.
- Handwriting may be difficult, so keyboarding skills are helpful.
- Reading/writing assignments should be kept as brief as possible to reduce stress and eye fatigue.
- Use of dark-line paper may be helpful.
- Directions and special words should be underlined.
- Attention should be paid to lighting and contrast.
- Window card with rectangular hole to view one word or line at a time may be useful for younger children.
- Telescope may be useful for distance vision tasks (watching television, street crossings, etc.).
- Student may benefit from counselling for adjustment to visual impairment.
- Vary tasks where possible to allow student a brief break from continuous reading.

Optic (Nerve) Atrophy

What is optic (nerve) atrophy?

Optic nerve atrophy is a condition where there is degeneration of nerve tissue which carries messages from the retina to the brain. Optic nerve atrophy may be caused by many factors and may develop in the pre-natal, peri-natal or post-natal period. Optic nerve atrophy may be progressive or stable and may affect both central and peripheral vision. The effects of this condition are very specific to individuals.

What are the characteristics of optic (nerve) atrophy?

- Decreased visual acuity.
- Peripheral or central field loss, depending on site of damage along the optic nerve.
- Colour vision may be impaired.
- Visual perception may be impaired.
- Fluctuating visual performance.

What are the functional implications of optic (nerve) atrophy?

- Glare must be avoided.
- Orientation and mobility skills will be of concern.
- Use of low vision aids may be helpful.
- Lighting will be a major factor in visual functioning.
- Depth perception may be affected.
- Student may have sensitivity to certain levels or types of light.

What are some educational considerations for a student with optic (nerve) atrophy?

- Student will need lighting considerations.
- Student may need extra time to complete visual tasks.
- Large print, high contrast and audio-taped materials may be helpful.
- Student may need to learn braille.

- Student may need to sit closer to the board or demonstrations.
- Student may need to use black felt pen or marker for writing.
- Student may need to use dark-lined paper.
- Avoid visual clutter.
- Student may benefit from breaks from visual tasks to combat eye fatigue.
- Glare should be avoided in all situations.
- Teacher needs to be aware that student's visual functioning may fluctuate, therefore, so should expectations.
- Student may benefit from use of low vision aids.
- Student will require orientation and mobility training.
- Keyboarding skills may be necessary.
- Student may need time to adjust to changes in lighting.
- Physical activity may be restricted; check with the student's ophthalmologist.

Ocular Albinism (ock-you-leral-bin-iz-um)

What is ocular albinism?

Ocular albinism is a hereditary deficiency of pigmentation which affects the retina and iris. Ocular albinism is commonly associated with high degrees of refractive error (near-sightedness and far-sightedness), nystagmus (involuntary motion of the eyes) and severe photophobia (sensitivity to light). Individuals with ocular albinism may or may not have pale skin and hair (oculocutaneous albinism).

What are the characteristics of ocular albinism?

- Decreased visual acuity.
- Nystagmus.
- Photophobia (extreme sensitivity to light).
- Eye fatigue when performing visual tasks.

What are the functional implications of ocular albinism?

- Orientation and mobility will be of concern.
- Training in daily living skills may be necessary.
- Glare must be avoided.
- Use of low vision aids may be helpful.
- Lighting will be a major factor in visual functioning.

What are some educational considerations for a student with ocular albinism?

- Student will need lighting considerations (normal to dim lighting may be preferable).
- Student may need extra time to complete tasks.
- Large print, high contrast and audio-taped materials may be helpful.
- Student may need to sit closer to the board or demonstrations.
- Student may need to use black felt pen or marker for writing.
- Student may need to use dark-lined paper.
- Training in the area of orientation and mobility may be necessary.
- Student may benefit from breaks from visual tasks to combat eye fatigue.
- Stress will complicate nystagmus, therefore assignments and writing tasks should be as brief as possible.
- Keyboarding skills will likely be important as students have difficulty with handwriting.
- Use of low vision aids may be helpful.
- Glare should be avoided in all situations.
- Student may benefit from a tilted reading stand.
- Student may need to use sunglasses or visors for light sensitivity.
- Student may need to learn organised search patterns to locate objects or visual targets.

- Training may be necessary in daily living skills.
- Student may benefit from adjustment to blindness counselling.
- Teacher should not stand in front of the window or other light source.

Retinal Detachment

What is retinal detachment?

Retinal detachment occurs when the parts of the retina pull away from the supporting structure of the eye and atrophy. Retinal detachment can be caused by diabetes, a blow to the head, trauma, breaks, holes or tears in the retina, degenerative myopia ('near-sightedness') or retinopathy of prematurity (ROP). Incidents of retinal detachment occur adventitiously (after birth) and the condition may be progressive or not. Immediate intervention may allow for surgical correction of the detachment so that there are no lasting effects on the vision. Immediate attention must be given to investigate symptoms of retinal detachment such as piercing pain in the eye, flash of light inside vision, field losses, increasing difficulty with night vision, multiple dark spots floating in the field of vision, distortion of colour vision, objects appearing smaller than normal or complaint of seeing a shadow or a curtain coming down or going up in the field of vision.

What are the characteristics of retinal detachment?

- Possible sudden, large changes in vision.
- Possible gradual, cumulative changes in vision which he or she may not notice.
- Student may need to restrict physical activities which could lead to head trauma.
- Night vision may be poor.
- Colour vision may be distorted.
- Visual fields or central vision may be affected.
- May accompany high myopia (near-sightedness).

What are the functional implications of retinal detachment?

- Use of certain low vision aids may be helpful.
- Lighting will be a major factor in visual functioning.
- Visual fatigue may be experienced when performing visual tasks.
- Student may complain of eyestrain.
- Performing visual tasks may cause headaches.

What are some educational considerations for a student with retinal detachment?

- Glare must be avoided.
- Student will need lighting considerations.
- Care must be taken to provide student with high contrast print materials.
- Student may need extra time to complete visual tasks.
- Student may need to sit closer to the board or demonstrations.
- Student may need assistance or alternate ways to take notes.
- Student may need to use black felt pen, marker and/or dark-line paper for writing.
- Student may benefit from breaks from visual tasks to combat eye fatigue.
- Student may require orientation and mobility training.
- Physical activities may need to be restricted; check with the student's ophthalmologist.
- Where possible, student should be given opportunities for manipulation of concrete objects instead of pencil and paper tasks.

Optic Nerve Hypoplasia (hi-po-play-shuh) (ONH)

What is optic nerve hypoplasia?

Optic nerve hypoplasia (ONH) is a condition in which there is incomplete development of the optic nerve. It may occur in one or both eyes and the visual loss is variable. ONH occurs in association with other developmental anomalies, fetal alcohol syndrome and substance abuse. Less severe and subtle cases may go undetected into adulthood. Vision loss associated with ONH is not progressive.

What are the characteristics of optic nerve hypoplasia?

- Possible nystagmus (uncontrolled movement of the eyes).
- Possible amblyopia ('lazy eye').
- Field loss is likely.
- Visual loss is variable.

What are the functional implications of optic nerve hypoplasia?

- Use of certain low vision aids may be helpful.
- Lighting may be a major factor in visual functioning.
- Visual fatigue may be experienced when performing visual tasks.
- Use of large print, high contrast materials may be helpful.
- Braille and tactual materials may be needed by some students.
- Student may have social interaction problems.

What are some educational considerations for a student with optic nerve hypoplasia?

- Glare must be avoided.
- Student will need lighting considerations.
- Visual clutter should be avoided.
- Teacher should avoid standing in front of a busy background and/or wearing clothing with busy patterns.
- Vision stimulation is essential for young children to help them learn to interpret what they see.
- Care must be taken to provide student with high contrast print materials.
- Student may need extra time to complete visual tasks.
- Student may need to sit closer to the board or demonstrations.

- Student may have difficulty with fine motor skills such as cutting paper, coloring or printing within lines.
- Line markers, line guides or rulers may help student keep place on the page.
- Student may need to use black felt pen or marker for writing.
- Reading/writing sessions may need to be kept as brief as possible to reduce eye fatigue.
- Tasks requiring depth perception such as catching a ball or moving in uneven terrain may be difficult.
- Mobility around school and playground may need to be monitored due to reduced depth perception.
- Preferential lighting may be considered.
- Glare should be avoided.
- Student may need familiarisation with the environment to help anticipate distances and heights.

Retinopathy (ret-in-ah-puh-thee) of Prematurity (ROP)

What is retinopathy of prematurity?

Retinopathy of prematurity (ROP) is a condition in which the blood vessels in the retina are improperly formed as a result of an infant being born prematurely and supplemental oxygen being given during the neonatal period. Because the infant is premature, blood vessels are not matured and hemorrhages in the retina occur. Also, scar tissue forms and newly developing blood vessels are abnormal. The incidence and severity of ROP is related to birth weight and gestational age. There may be minimal, temporary damage or permanent and total blindness. Early laser surgery to prevent the progression of the disease is sometimes necessary. This condition used to be referred to as 'retrolental fibroplasia'.

What are the characteristics of retinopathy of prematurity?

- Decreased visual acuity.
- At higher risk for retinal detachment.

- Possible severe myopia (near-sightedness).
- Spotty vision.
- Strabismus (eyes not straight) or amblyopia ('lazy eye').
- Retinal scarring.
- Field loss.
- Possible glaucoma

What are the functional implications of retinopathy of prematurity?

- Early intervention is crucial.
- Sensory stimulation through lots of experiences is crucial.
- Low contact sports and leisure activities should be considered.
- Orientation and mobility may be of concern, especially spatial skills.
- Training in daily living skills may be necessary.
- Glare must be avoided.
- Use of low vision aids may be helpful.
- Lighting will be a major factor in visual functioning.
- Often, low birth weight children have increased social problems, learning disabilities and socialisation problems.

What are some educational considerations for student with retinopathy of prematurity?

- Student will need high levels of lighting.
- Large print, high contrast and audio-taped materials may be helpful.
- Student may need to learn braille.
- Student may need to use black felt pen or marker for writing.
- Student may need to use dark-lined paper.
- Training in the area of orientation and mobility will be crucial.

There will likely be questions from other students about your child's visual impairment.

Have you any suggestions about what might be said and how it should be presented in class?

____

____

____

Are there any other people working with your child that I should know about?

____

____

What educational and social goals do you have for your child?

____

____

Are there any other questions you would like to ask me? For example: what are my classroom expectations; assignments; materials; activities; and assessments of progress, projects, portfolios or tests?

____

____

What specialised equipment does your child use at home and at school (Braille 'n Speak, braille printer, CCTV)?

____

____

Appendix G

Information from an Education Consultant or Itinerant

Teacher/Strategist for Students with Visual Impairments.

To help provide appropriate programming, please provide the following information:

Degree and Nature of Visual Impairment

An explanation of the student's visual impairment:

____

____

An explanation of the student's use of residual vision in the classroom:

____

____

____

Educational and Social Needs

What equipment should be used? How is it obtained by the school?

____

____

____

Index

A

Accessibility/ Infrastructure for Disability
..initiatives , 134-35
..intervention required, 136
Achromatopsia (Eye Condition), 183
ADIP Scheme (for Assistance in Purchasing Aids), 159
Aids & Appliances
..(ADIP Scheme for purchase), 159
..distribution to CWSN, 80
Ali Yavar Jung National Institute for the Hearing Handicapped, 152
...objectives, 153
All India Confederation of the Blind- Study on Blindness
Compensatory Skills, 85
Amblyopia, 189-90
Aniridia (Eye Condition), 185
Anthropophagic/ Anthropoemic strategy, 28-29
Assistive Technology, 98, 105
..issues & challenges, 114
..Training need, 117
..accessibility to educational software, 119
Astigmatism, 188-89
Audio Supported Reading - benefits, 106

B

Blind/ Visually Impaired schools - India - History/ accounts, 54-55
Blindness Rehabilitation, 32
Blindness, 40
conditions, 40
effects, 40, 42
problems, 41
distribution/causes, 46
Braille Codes -India, 110
Braille in India Advent, 109
Braille
Embosser, 111
Keyboards, 112
Translator Software, 110

Writer, 107

C

Cascade Model
(Deno's), 59
Cataracts, 186-87
Closed Circuit TV, 112
Coloboma, 202-204
Computational Aids, 108
Computter Use (Blind)
approaches, 112-13
Conceptual Model of
Special Education, 59
Concessions (Govt)
for the Blind, 160-62
Conflicts Perspective of
disability, 27
critique, 27
Constitution of India
Provision for Disableds, 150
Convention on the Rights
of Persons with
Disabilities & its Optional
Protocol-UN-2006, 140
Cooley's Looking Glass Self, 27
Core Curriculum, 93
..existing, 93
.. expanded, 94
..significance, 99
Cortical Visual Impairment, 191-92
Curriculum of Visually
Impaired, 89
Existing, 93
Suggestions, 100, 102
Unique needs, 101
assessment, 89
in pre-school, 90
Elementary Secondary
Level, 92
CWD identification/
inconsistencies, 72
CWSN identification/
definition, 72-73
CWSN integration in
Regular schools, 165
CWSN distribution of
aids/appliances, 80

D

Decisions for disabled
critique- Finklestein, 31
Deen Dayal Disabled
Rehabilitation Scheme, 150
Development Milestones for
Infants with Visual
impairment, 179-80
Disability
Definition, 15, 22
DFID on, 15
Nature, 15
Numbers (NSSO-2002), 71
Notions/Models
/Approach, 16, 39
linguistic meaning, 39
Rights - Legislation, 75
Disability-wise Segregation
of Population, 71
Disabled friendly
Buses, 133
Environment
- promotion, 131
Discriminating disableds, 26
Discrimination of Disabled
(Prohibition) in employment, 147
District Disability and
Rehabilitation Centre (DDRC), 67
Durkheim, Emile
on pre/post industrialization
societies, 25
Education of Disabled, 49
International scene, 49

efforts- India, 63

E

Educational Barriers, 69-70
Educational Consultant
(information from), 227-28
Electronic Equipment
(assisting Visually
Impaired), 107
Elementary and Secondary
Levels Blinds
curriculum, 92
Embossed Braille Paper, 108
Employment Exchange
for the Disabled, 140
Employment Rate
of the Disabled, 141
..fall-reasons, 140-41
Enrolment in schools
of the disableds, 73
Environmental awareness, 96

F

File Review Form, 222
Four Track Tape recorder, 112
Functional Perspective
of Disability, 25
... Farber on, 25
Fundamental Rights, 57

G

Gaze manifestations
- Foucalt, Sartre, 29
Concept, 30
impact, 30
Gender Inequities
of Disableds, 75
Glaucoma, 194-95
GPS System, 106-107
Graphing Aids, 108
Haptic Devices, 112
Hemianopsia, 193-94
Human Rights Approach
to disability, 27

H

Hyperopia, 198

I

Identification of disableds, 72
Identifying Children with
disabilities, 163
IEDS Scheme, 77
Inclusive Education
Principles, 65
for disableds-India, 65
Action Plan, 66
Individual Approach of
Disability, 16, 20
...criticism, 18
Institute for the Physically
Handicapped- New Delhi, 156
Institutes for PWDs, 151
Institutional Approach, 31
Integrated Education for
Children at Secondary
Stage(IEDSS), 67
Integrated Education for
the Disabled Children(IEDC),
66
Integrated Education Scheme
for the Disabled Children, 162
Integrated Education Schools
critique, 81
Integrated Education(India)
Limitations/ Deficiencies, 79
NPE on, 61
emergence, 62
for Visualy impaired, 62
Integrated/Segregated
Plan(Deno's), 59
schools, 63
Integration of Disableds, 57
Programmes

..aspects, 58
..trends, 61
International Classification of Impairments, Disabilities and Handicaps (ICIDH)-WHO, 18
Interview With Parents, 224

L

Language teaching, 101
Leber's Optic atrophy, 196-98
Legislation Process & Policies
..critique, 140
..enforcement restrictions -factors, 142
Legislations for Disableds, 139
Legislations for PWEDs, 150-51
Literacy Figures of disableds, 145
Long Cane, 114
Low Vision Aids, 109
Low Vision, 42
- Distribution/causes, 46

M

Macular Degeneration, 201-202
Mathematical Aids, 109
Mathematics
teaching of, 100
Medical & Social Models
difference, 37
Medical Certificate - Vision, 220-21
Medical Models-Disability , 16, 18-19
Mobility Skills, 95-96
Myopia, 199
Mystery of the Eye
and Shadow of Blindness, 32

N

National Awards for the Welfare of Persons With Disabilities, 159
National Centre for Promotion of Employment of Disabled People (NCPEDP)Survey-1999, 145
National Handicapped Finance and Development Corporation, 160
National Institute for Empowerment of Persons with Multiple Disabilities - Chennai ...objectives, 157-58
National Institute for the Orthopaedically Handicapped- Kolkata, 155
National Institute for the Visually Handicapped -Dehradun, 151
National Institute of Open Schooling, 84
National Institute of Rehabilitation Training & Research- Cuttack, 155
National Policy on Education (NPE) on Integrated Education, 61
National Scholarship Schemes of PWDs, 158
Nomad Pad, 111
Non-electronic Equipment (assisting Visually Impaired), 107
Nystagmus, 204-205

O

Ocular Albinism, 207
Oliver, Mike
on disability, 22-23
Oppression of Disabled, 37
Optic Nerve Atrophy, 206-207
Optic Nerve Hypoplasia, 210-11
Orientation and Mobility
Skills, 95
Aids, 113

P

Pedestrian Environment
for Disabled, 132
features/problems, 132, 135
Personal Tragedy Theory, 16
criticism, 18
Persons With Disabilities (PWD) Equal Opportunities Protection of Rights and Full Participation Act, 1995, 39, 113, 117, 130
Political Approach to Disability, 26
Portable Note takers, 111
Portable Reading Devices, 106
Post - Modernist Perspective of Disability, 28
Pre-School Blind
Curriculum, 90-91
...points to consider, 91
Projected Integrated Education for the Disableds(PIED)
critique, 69
PSUs employing disabled, 142
Psychological Model
- disability, 17
PWD Act-1995, 83, 144-45, 147
PWD Placements
through Employmnnt Exchanges, 144
PWD Reserved Posts
-2003, 143

Q

Quota Policy for Disabled, 143

R

Recreation/Leisure Skills, 98
Rehabilitation of
Visually Impaired, 149
Strategies, 149
Reservation for Disabled, 142
Residential Schools for
Disabled, 49-50
..services, 50-51
..definition, 51
..role, characteristics, 51
Visually Impaired- India, 54
..history, 54
Response to Intervention
Model(RIT)-Education, 52
Retinal Detachment, 209
Retinitis Pigmentosa, 213
Retinoblastoma, 212-13
Retinopathy of
Prematurity, 216-17
Road transport accesibility
for disabled, 133
Rogers Teachers /
Student Centered Approach, 123

S

Sartre on Gaze, 29
Scanners (OCR), 112
School Observation Checklist
issues, 83
on educational aids, 84
Schools Enrollment in
Integrated Educational
Program Primary
/Upper Primary, 78
Science & Technology
Project in Mission Mode, 160
Science teaching, 101
Screen Readers
(Text to Speech), 111
Screen Reading Software, 106, 111
Self- Independence Skills, 97
Self Protection Techniques, 97
Sewell Raised-Line
Drawing Kit, 108

Signages
provision / efforts, 135
Slate and stylus, 107
Social Approach of
disability, 20, 23
Oliver on, 23
Theoretical perspectives, 25
criticism, 35
Social Skills, 97
Social Studies
teaching, 101
Societies
negative role, 31
Sonic Pathfinder, 114
Special Education for
Disabled Children
-trends, 53
-rural/urban, 53
Speech Synthesisers, 111
Stigma
Goffman on, 28
Strabismus(squint), 215
Symptoms checklist
for Teachers
(Visual Problems), 181-82
Systems (different)
observation of disabilities, 33
Systems Model, 32
levels of Social Systems, 33-34

T

Taylor Slate, 108
Teachers Attitude
towards mainstreaming, 124
Teachers
Role/Approach, 121-25
overview, 125
The Two in One : Walking
With Smokie, Walking
With Blindness, 32
Topliss
on discriminaion of PWDs, 26
Transactional Model, 34
Travel Concessions, 160-61

U

Urban Development Ministry
.. Planning for Disabled, 131
Urban/Rural enrolment
of disableds, 77
Usher Syndrome, 218

V

Visual disability
NSSO definition, 39
Visual Impairment
Prevalence, 43
NSSO on, 44
Age Groups, 44
Onset, 45..age, 45
Visually Handicapped Students
Schools
..hurdles, 83
..infrastructure, 84
Visually Impaired
barriers to education, 82
Visually Impaired
Figures WHO-2009, 116
Voluntary Organizations
in Integrated Education, 77

W

Welfare Programmes
Schemes for PWDs, 158